Multiple Sclerosis

Edited by Stavros J. Baloyannis

Published in London, United Kingdom

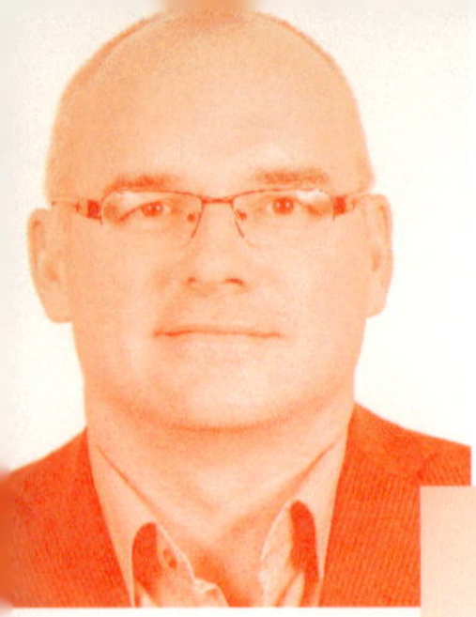
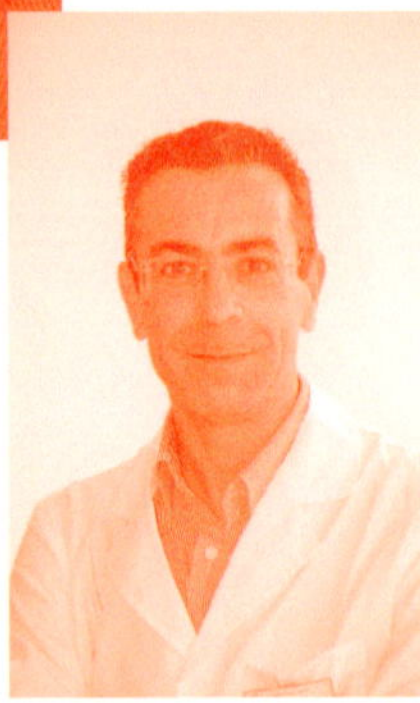
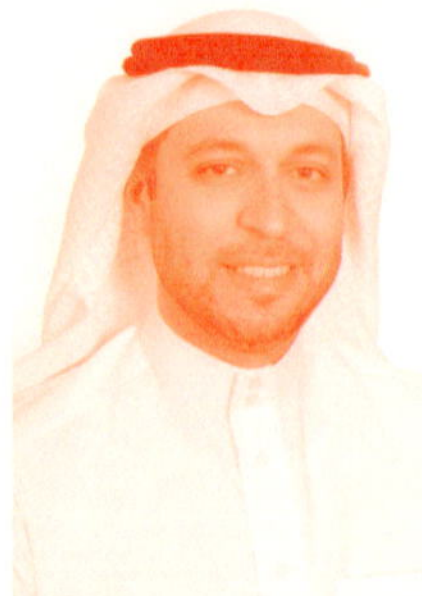
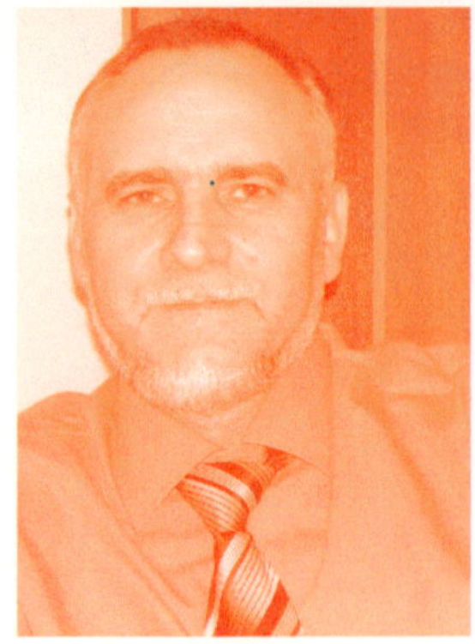
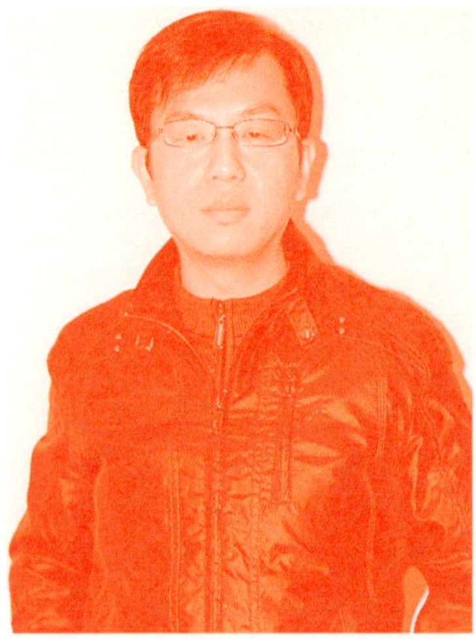
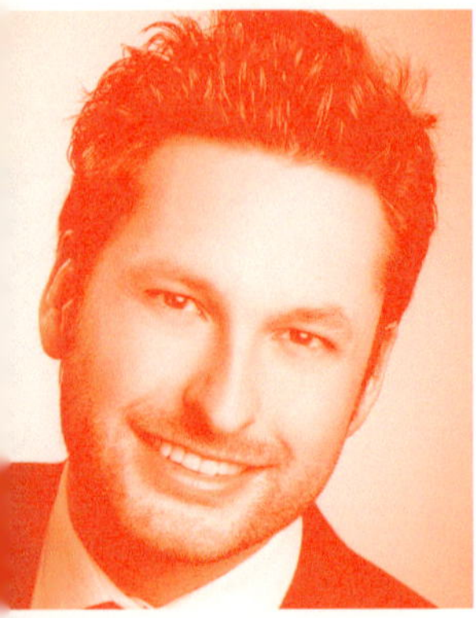
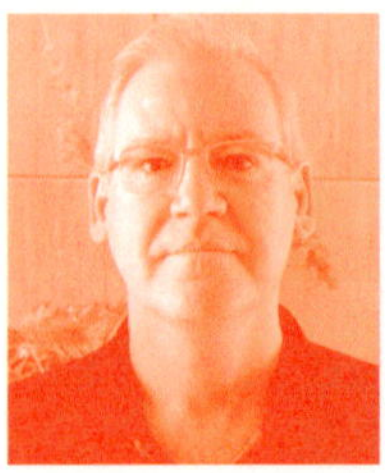

IntechOpen

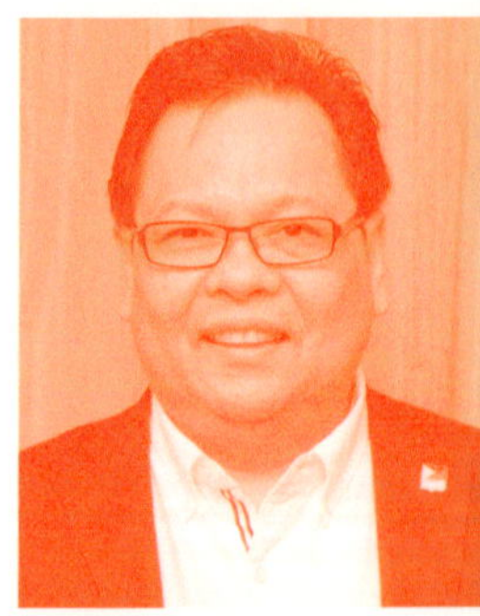
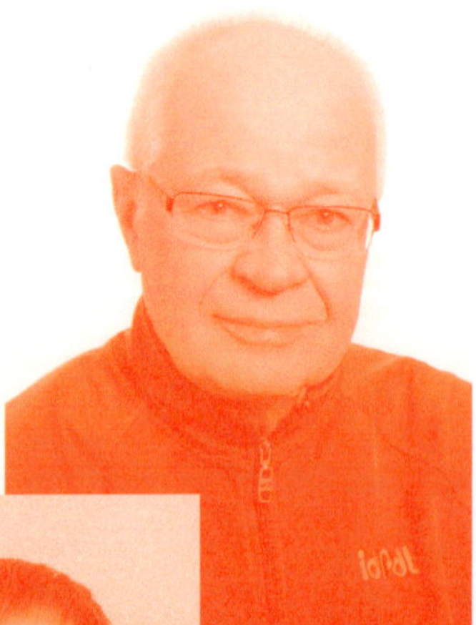
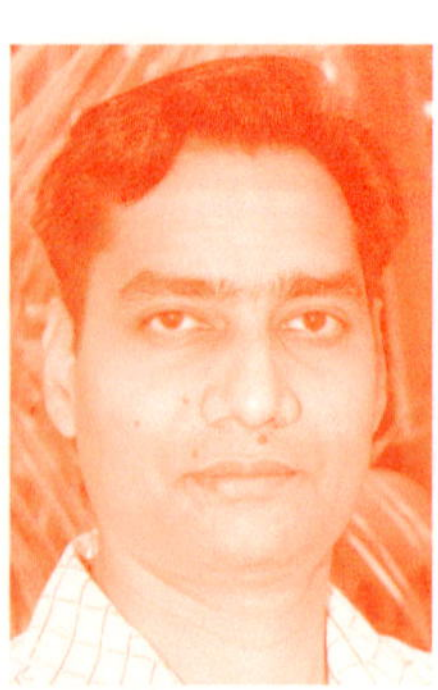
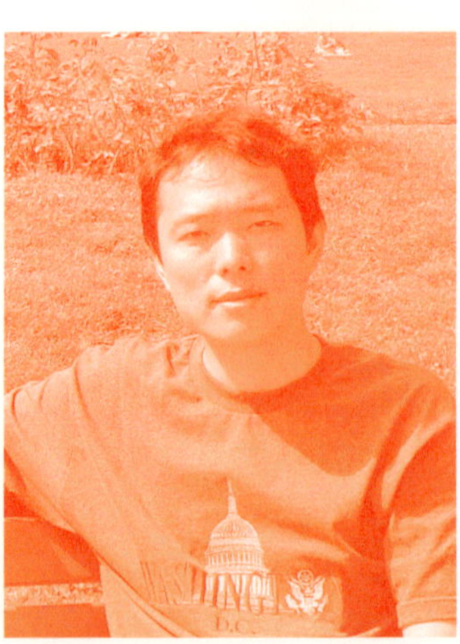
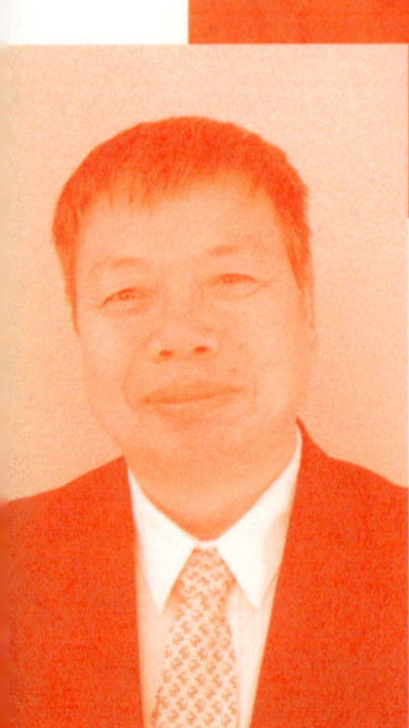
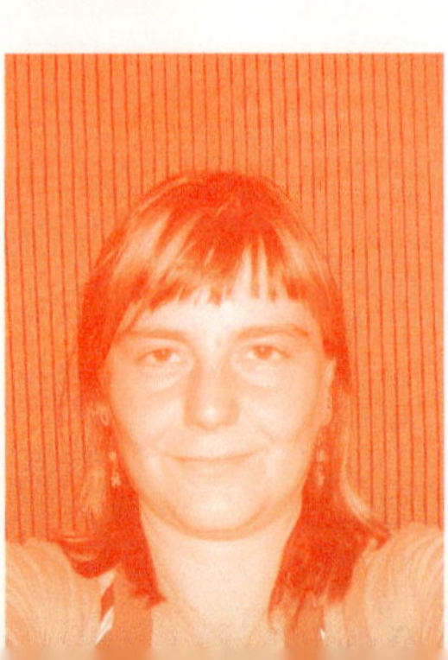

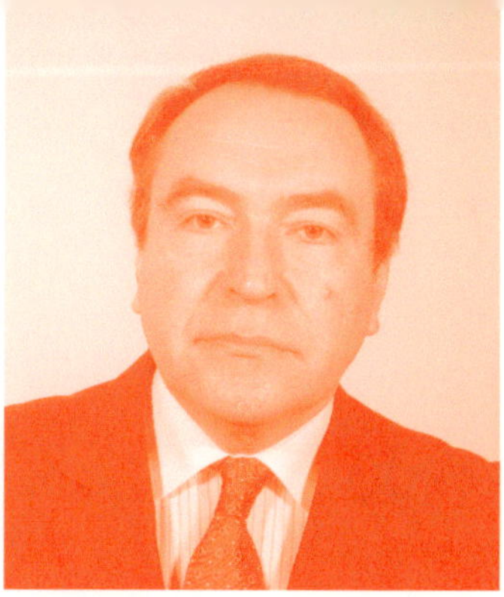
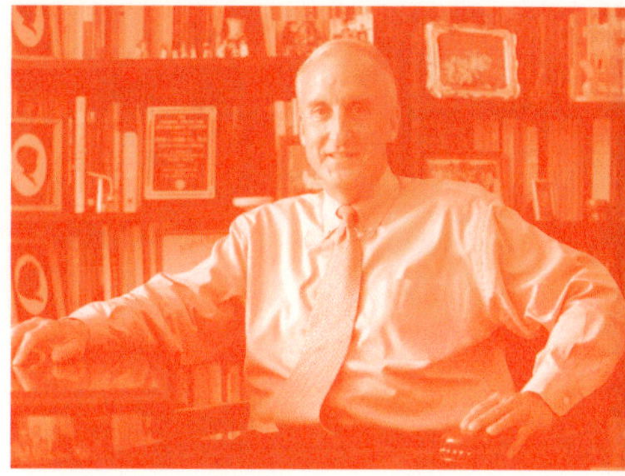
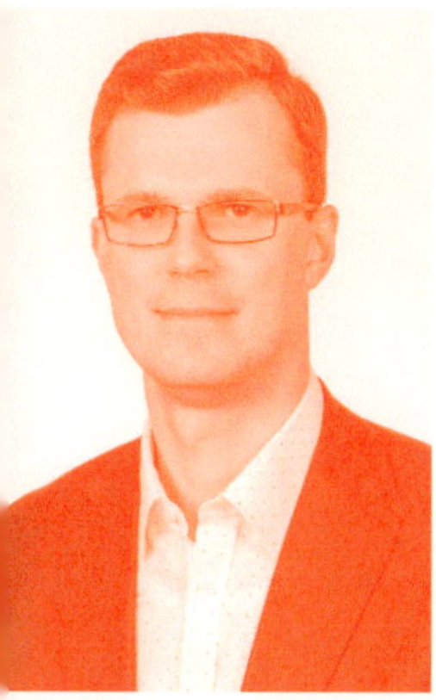
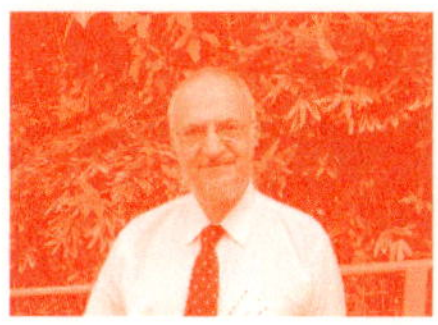
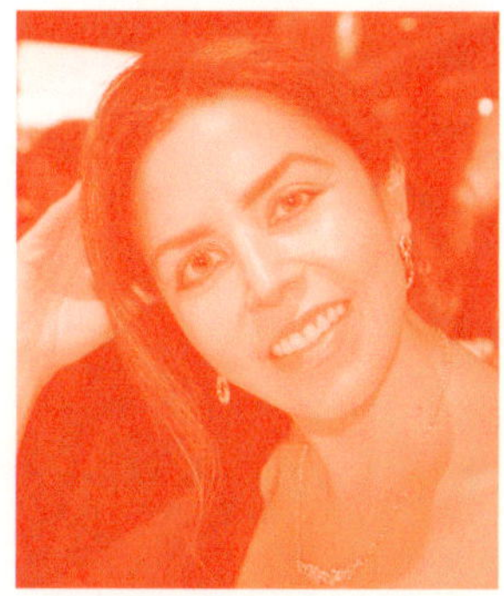

Supporting open minds since 2005

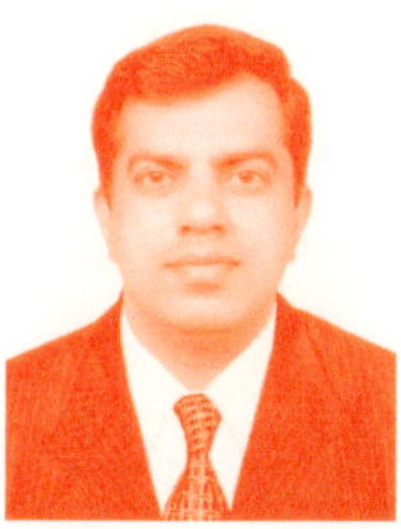
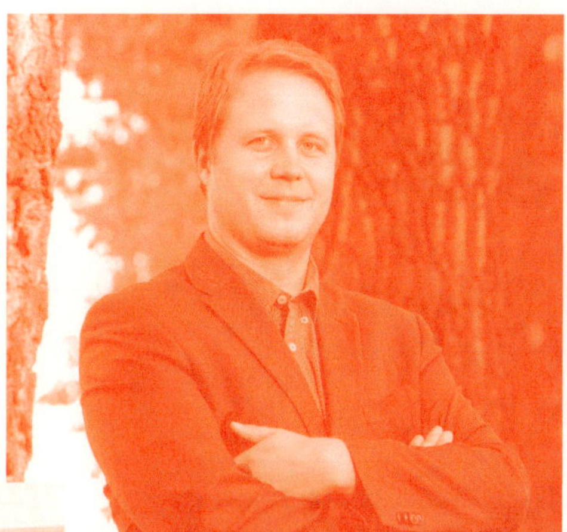
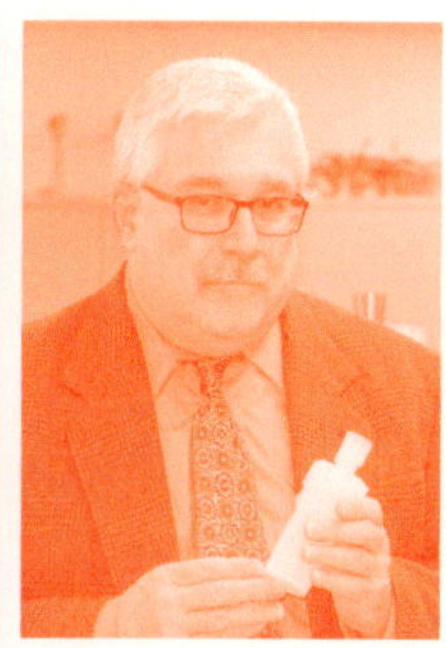
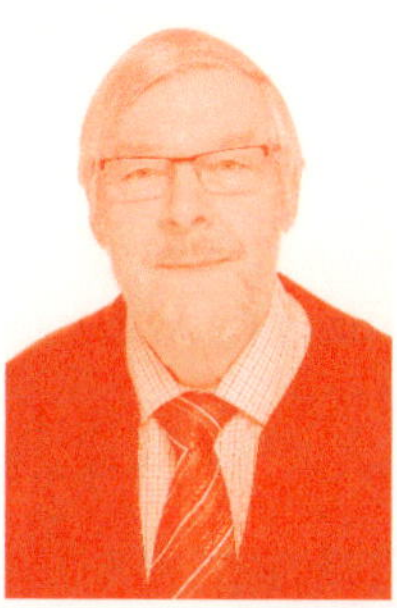
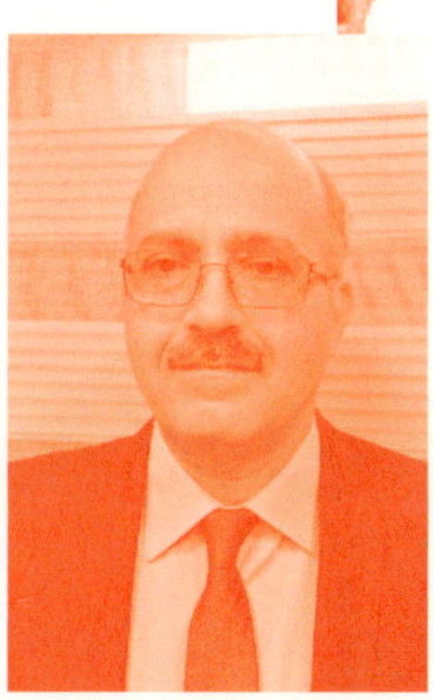
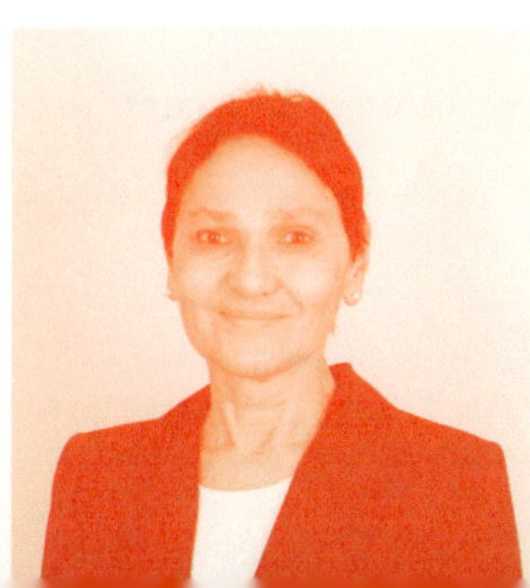
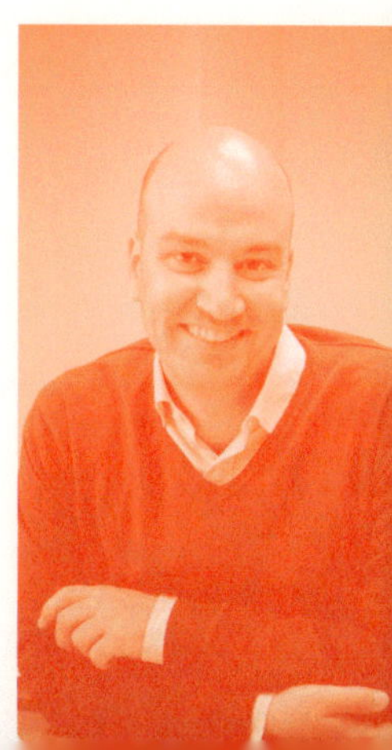

Multiple Sclerosis
http://dx.doi.org/10.5772/intechopen.78425
Edited by Stavros J. Baloyannis

Contributors
Joyce Pauline Joseph, Majid Soltani, Athena Soulika, Nagendra Rai, Marilyn Wang, Sofia Caryotakis, Alan Nguyen, Gulfaraz Khan, Asma Hassani, Lambros Messinis, Panagiotis Papathanasopoulos, Grigorios Nasios, Seyyedeh Zahra Safi, Stavros J Baloyannis

First published in London, United Kingdom, 2020 by IntechOpen
IntechOpen is the global imprint of INTECHOPEN LIMITED, registered in England and Wales, registration number: 11086078, 7th floor, 10 Lower Thames Street, London, EC3R 6AF, United Kingdom
Printed in Croatia

British Library Cataloguing-in-Publication Data
A catalogue record for this book is available from the British Library

Additional hard and PDF copies can be obtained from orders@intechopen.com

Multiple Sclerosis
Edited by Stavros J. Baloyannis
p. cm.
Print ISBN 978-1-78984-331-6
Online ISBN 978-1-78984-332-3
eBook (PDF) ISBN 978-1-83968-557-6

For EU product safety concerns:
IN TECH d.o.o., Prolaz Marije Krucifikse Kozulić 3, 51000 Rijeka, Croatia, info@intechopen.com or visit our website at intechopen.com.

Meet the editor

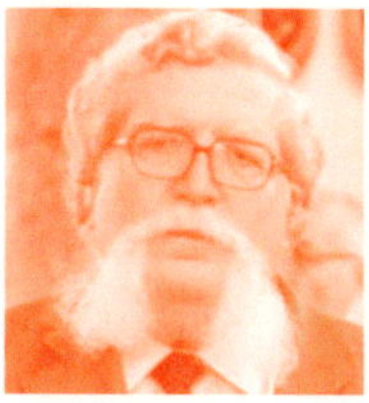

Stavros J. Baloyannis, Professor Emeritus of Neurology at Aristotelian University, Thessaloniki, Greece, was born in Thessaloniki. He graduated from the School of Medicine, Aristotelian University. He trained in neurology at Aristotelian University and the Institute of Neurology, London, neuropathology at the Institute of Neurology, London, Catholic University of Louvain, and University of Pennsylvania, neuropathology of auditory pathways at Harvard University, electron microscopy at the University of Pennsylvania, and neuroimmunology at Yale University. His research includes the blood–brain barrier, mitochondria in Alzheimer's disease, synaptogenesis, neuronal apoptosis, dendritic and synaptic pathology, and Golgi apparatus in dementias. His special interests are neuroethics, neurolinguistics, neurophilosophy, and the history of neurosciences, neurology, and art. He is a member of 60 scientific societies, and an honorary member of the Academy of Hellenic Air Forces, President of the Society for the Amelioration of the Quality of Life in Chronic Neurological Diseases, President of the Orthodox Association for Medical Education and Health in Africa, and visiting professor at Tufts University, Democritus University, Aristotelian University, School of Theology, and School of Philosophy. He is the author of 28 textbooks and 723 papers on neurology and neurosciences. He has organized 26 international congresses and participated in 612 world congresses on neurology, neuropathology, psychiatry, and medical ethics. He is the author of two books of poems. He was head of the Department of Neurology at Aristotelian University (1992–2011) and Director of Research Institute for Alzheimer's Disease.

Contents

Preface

Multiple sclerosis (MS) has for years been a crucial unsolved problem in the field of neurosciences, and is a serious cause of suffering for millions of patients worldwide, affecting psychosomatic homeostasis in the majority of patients.

The etiopathological background of the disease, which is presumably a progressive inflammation of the central nervous system (CNS), inducing demyelination in the white matter and degenerative alterations in the gray matter, provoking a multitude of polymorphic clinical phenomena, is still an open field of intensive, constantly progressive investigation.

The incidence of MS varies across geographic regions, with high rates in high latitude, affecting three times more women than men at any age. Many genetic factors, major histocompatibility complex and non-major histocompatibility complex, may play an important role in the innate immune mechanisms and in the modulation of the immune system under the influence of the many exterior environmental risk factors and viral infections.

A large number of patients have from the onset experienced relapses and remissions of various neurological phenomena, lasting for many years, whereas a substantial number of untreated patients face the tragedy of continuous deterioration of their physical and mental condition, resulting in a serious irreversible disability.

Energy failure is the substantial cause of functional impairment in the majority of patients who suffer from MS. That cause is reasonably associated with neuronal degeneration, demyelination, and axonal loss based on a wide spectrum of innate autoimmune mechanisms, inflammatory reactions, mitochondrial dysfunction, cytokine interactions, intracellular and interstitial edema, and perivascular cell reactions.

The clinical manifestations of the disease vary from person to person, from time to time, and from age to age, and most of them are changeable in the majority of the cases even from the initial stages of the disease. Vertigo, nausea, vomiting, hiccups, motor deficits, tremors, dysarthria, cutaneous sensory deficits, sensory phenomena from mucosae, cerebellar dysfunction, gait instability, diplopia, vision impairment, visual field defects, dyschromatopsia, phosphenes, painful conditions, autonomic dysfunction, sphincter insufficiency, fatigue, and cognitive decline, such as episodic memory deficits and impaired visuospacial estimation, emerging early in the disease compose a part of the resizing pattern of the disease. Cognitive decline, which would be attributed to association of gray and white matter lesions, in addition to disconnection and dissociation syndrome, is frequently underestimated in the initial stages of the disease, necessitating neuropsychological evaluation by properly designed tools for MS patients. Cognitive rehabilitation, which is essential for the improvement of the quality of life of patients, may include various methods and techniques enabling patients to overcome common problems of everyday life, coping harmoniously with the disease burden. Language disorders are not rare phenomena in patients who suffer from MS, necessitating appropriate speech therapy.

Diagnostic criteria for MS have been proposed and introduced for many years, and have been revised many times. Most of them may simply facilitate the approach of the diagnosis of the disease. Among them, diffusion imaging, resting state functional magnetic resonance imaging, magnetic resonance spectroscopy, evoked potentials, optical coherence tomography (OCT), OCT angiography, and immunological analysis of the cerebrospinal fluid may lead to a prompt diagnosis of the disease even in patients with atypical clinical manifestations and course heterogeneity.

However, in the differential diagnoses of MS a substantial number of other conditions mimicking the clinical manifestations of the disease should be under consideration. Among them neuromyelitis optica spectrum disorder (Devic's disease) would be differentially diagnosed on the basis of anti-aquaporin 4 antibody, acute disseminated encephalomyelitis on the basis of the clinical profile and neuroimaging data, myelin oligodendrocyte glycoprotein (MOG) antibody disease on the basis of the level of MOG antibodies, and antiphospholipid syndrome by the detection of lupus anticoagulant and anticardiolipin antibodies. In addition, systemic lupus erythematosus, small vessel disease, and Susac's syndrome have also a place in the expanded spectrum of the differential diagnosis of MS.

There is no definite targeted therapeutic approach for MS. An efficient therapeutic strategy should be based on clear knowledge of the pathogenetic mechanisms of the disease. Investigation of the role of myeloid cells and the infiltration of the CNS by peripheral lymphoid and myeloid cells may be crucial for a deeper understanding of the progression of the disease and the chronicity of the clinical phenomena. Novel therapeutic attempts aimed at modulating the activities and reactions of myeloid cells might be hopeful in treating MS patients at the initial stages of the disease. In addition, the application of autologous Epstein-Barr virus-specific T cell therapy may improve the clinical condition of patients. Non-pharmacological therapies, such as appropriate diet, proper environment, physical exercise, relaxation and progressive muscle relaxation therapy, psychotherapy, cognitive behavioral therapy, music therapy, and emotional, social, and spiritual support may also play a beneficial role in the amelioration of the quality of life in the large majority of patients.

In this volume, the authors discuss some of the crucial aspects of the MS drama, attempting to contribute to finding a way that may lead to catharsis.

Stavros J. Baloyannis MD, PhD
Professor Emeritus,
Aristotelian University,
Thessaloniki, Greece

Section 1

Introduction

Chapter 1

Introductory Chapter: Multiple Sclerosis

Stavros J. Baloyannis

1. In the labyrinth of multiple sclerosis

Multiple sclerosis (MS) remains a crucial unsolved problem in the field of neurosciences, being also a serious cause of suffering for millions of patients worldwide affecting the quality of life, the personal and social economy, and the psychosomatic homeostasis substantially in the majority of the patients.

The etiopathological background of the disease, which is a progressive inflammation of the CNS [1, 2], inducing demyelination in the white matter and degenerative alterations in the gray matter in various areas of the brain hemispheres, the cerebellum, the brain stem, and the spinal cord, may provoke a multitude of polymorphic clinical phenomena inducing a variable type of physical, mental, and social disability in the suffering people [3, 4].

The incidence of MS varies considerably across geographic regions, with high rates in high latitude and low in the tropical zone, affecting three times more women than men at any age, though the climax is between 20 and 40 years. Approximately 2.5 million people in the world suffer from multiple sclerosis nowadays, and 700,000 among them are registered in Europe [5–7].

Many genetic factors, MHC and non-MHC, may play an important role in the innate immune mechanisms and in the modulation of the immune system under the influence of the many exterior environmental risk factors and viral infections [8, 9]. Among the viruses, the infection with Epstein–Barr virus (EBV), which is a common human herpes virus, seems to have a considerable association with the incidence of MS, particularly among pediatric patients [10–12].

A large number of patients have from onset the experience of relapses and remissions of the various neurological phenomena, lasting for many years, whereas a substantial number of untreated patients face the tragedy of the continuous deterioration of their physical and mental condition, resulting in a serious irreversible disability eventually, though primary progressive forms starting from the onset of the disease may also occur in approximately 10–15% of patients [13, 14].

Energy failure is obviously the substantial cause of the functional impairment in the majority of patients who suffer from multiple sclerosis. That cause is reasonably associated with demyelination, neuronal degeneration, and axonal loss, based on a wide spectrum of innate autoimmune mechanisms, inflammatory reactions, mitochondrial dysfunction, cytokine interactions, intracellular and interstitial edema, and perivascular cell reactions [15, 16].

2. The multiform suffering

The multiform clinical manifestations of the disease vary from person to person, from time to time, from age to age, and most of them are unstable and changeable in the majority of the cases even from the initial stages of the disease. Vertigo, nausea, vomiting, hiccups, motor deficits, tremors, dysarthria, cutaneous sensory deficits, sensory phenomena from mucosae, cerebellar dysfunction, gait instability, diplopia, vision impairment, visual field defects, dyschromatopsia, phosphenes, hearing impairment, painful conditions, neuralgia of the trigeminal nerve, autonomic dysfunction, sphincter insufficiency, fatigue, and cognitive decline, such as episodic memory deficits and impaired visuospacial estimation, emerging early in the disease compose a part of the frequently resizing pattern of the disease [17].

Particularly, cognitive decline, which would be attributed to the association of gray and white matter lesions [18], in addition to disconnection and dissociation syndrome, is frequently underestimated in the initial stages of the disease, necessitating neuropsychological evaluation by properly designed tools for MS patients [19]. In fact, cognitive phenomena are evident in the same degree of severity during all the stages of the disease, concerning all clinical subtypes [20, 21]. Cognitive rehabilitation, which is essential for the improvement of the quality of life of the patients, may include various methods and technics enabling the patients to overcome common problems of everyday life and to cope harmoniously with the disease burden, improving skills and capacities on the basis of the neuronal plasticity and the principle of functional reorganization of the brain [22, 23].

Language disorders are not rare phenomena in patients who suffer from MS [24]. The naming deficit, semantic paraphasia, impaired verbal fluency, grammar and syntax deficits, and the loss of high-level language skills necessitate the appropriate speech therapy [25].

3. Searching for the truth

Diagnostic criteria for multiple sclerosis have been proposed and introduced for many years and have been revised over times [26]. Most of them may simply facilitate the approach of the diagnosis of the disease. In general, the clinical estimation of the patients and the incorporation of data from the paraclinical investigation, especially from MRI [27], diffusion imaging, resting state functional MRI, magnetic resonance spectroscopy, evoked potentials, optical coherence tomography (OCT) [28], OCT angiography, and immunological analysis of the CSF, may lead to a prompt diagnosis of the disease even in patients with atypical clinical manifestations and marked course heterogeneity [29, 30].

In the cases that clinical and neuroimaging data are atypical or inadequate for posing the diagnosis of MS, the findings of oligoclonal band and immunoglobulin G (IgG) level in the cerebrospinal fluid analysis, in correlation with the serum data, would be a strong argument of intrathecal inflammation, advocating in favor of the diagnosis of MS [31].

However, in the differential diagnosis of multiple sclerosis, a substantial number of other conditions mimicking the clinical manifestations of the disease should be under consideration [32]. Among them, the neuromyelitis optica spectrum disorder (Devic's disease) would be differentially diagnosed on the basis of anti-aquaporin 4 antibody (AQP4-IgG) [33], the acute disseminated encephalomyelitis (ADEM) on the basis of the clinical profile and the neuroimaging data [34], the MOG antibody disease on the basis of the level of MOG antibodies [35], and the antiphospholipid syndrome by the detection of lupus anticoagulant and anticardiolipin antibodies [36]. In addition systemic lupus erythematosus, small vessel disease, and Susac's syndrome have a substantial place in the expanded spectrum of the differential diagnosis of MS [37].

Disease activity is usually estimated by the clinical relapses and the MRI findings of contrast-enhanced lesions, enabling the detection of new lesions on T2-weighted images. However, a reasonable criticism and a periodic reevaluation of the adopted diagnostic criteria would be of substantial importance for the accuracy of the prompt diagnosis of MS [38, 39].

4. Perspectives on resolution

There is no definite targeted therapeutic approach for MS [40–42]. The application of many current treatments aims at ameliorating the quality of life of the patients by reducing the disability progression and stabilizing the clinical condition of the patients [43].

The introduction of interferon in 1993 opened the horizons of many potential therapeutic options of various efficacy and side effects, which turned to raise many reasonable controversies from the viewpoint of the heterogeneity of the disease, the obscure etiopathological background, and the complexity of the pathophysiological mechanisms [44].

An efficient therapeutic strategy should be based on a clear knowledge of the pathogenetic mechanisms of the disease. The investigation of the role of the myeloid cells and the infiltration of the CNS by peripheral lymphoid and myeloid cells may be crucial for a deeper understanding of the progression of the disease and the chronicity of the clinical phenomena [45, 46].

Novel therapeutical attempts aiming at modulating the activities and reactions of myeloid cells might be hopeful in treating MS patients at the initial stages of the disease. In addition the application of autologous EBV-specific T cell therapy may improve the clinical condition of the patients, ameliorating consequently the quality of life in a substantial number of them [47–49].

Non-pharmacological therapies [50], such as appropriate diet [51], proper environment, physical exercise [52], psychological relaxation [53] and progressive muscle relaxation therapy (PMRT), psychotherapy [54], cognitive behavioral therapy [55], music therapy [56], and emotional, social, and spiritual support [57] may also play a considerable beneficial role in the amelioration of the quality of life in the large majority of the patients.

Author details

Stavros J. Baloyannis[1,2]

1 Aristotelian University of Thessaloniki, Thessaloniki, Greece

2 Research Institute for Neurodegenerative Diseases, Heraklion, Lagada, Greece

*Address all correspondence to: sibh844@otenet.gr

References

[1] Carroll M. Innate immunity in the etiopathology of autoimmunity. Nature Immunology. 2001;**2**(12):1089

[2] Tiwari S, Lapierre J, Ojha CR, Martins K, Parira T, Dutta RK, et al. Signaling pathways and therapeutic perspectives related to environmental factors associated with multiple sclerosis. Journal of Neuroscience Research. 2018;**96**(12):1831-1846

[3] Marrie RA, Patten SB, Berrigan LI, Tremlett H, Wolfson C, Warren S, et al. Diagnoses of depression and anxiety versus current symptoms and quality of life in multiple sclerosis. International Journal of MS Care. 2018;**20**(2):76-84

[4] Malivoire BL, Hare CJ, Hart TL. Psychological symptoms and perceived cognitive impairment in multiple sclerosis: The role of rumination. Rehabilitation Psychology. 2018;**63**(2):286

[5] Browne P, Chandraratna D, Angood C, Tremlett H, Baker C, Taylor BV, et al. Atlas of multiple sclerosis 2013: A growing global problem with widespread inequity. Neurology. 2014;**83**(11):1022-1024

[6] Kingwell E, Marriott JJ, Jetté N, Pringsheim T, Makhani N, Morrow SA, et al. Incidence and prevalence of multiple sclerosis in Europe: A systematic review. BMC Neurology. 2013;**13**(1):128

[7] Koutsouraki E, Costa V, Baloyannis S. Epidemiology of multiple sclerosis in Europe: A review. International Review of Psychiatry. 2010;**22**(1):2-13

[8] Lutton JD, Winston R, Rodman TC. Multiple sclerosis: Etiological mechanisms and future directions. Experimental Biology and Medicine. 2004;**229**(1):12-20

[9] Axisa PP, Hafler DA. Multiple sclerosis: Genetics, biomarkers, treatments. Current Opinion in Neurology. 2016;**29**(3):345-353

[10] Jons D, Sundström P, Andersen O. Targeting Epstein-Barr virus infection as an intervention against multiple sclerosis. Acta Neurologica Scandinavica. 2015;**131**(2):69-79

[11] Garg N, Smith TW. An update on immunopathogenesis, diagnosis, and treatment of multiple sclerosis. Brain and Behavior: A Cognitive Neuroscience Perspective. 2015;**5**(9):e00362

[12] Fernández-Menéndez S, Fernández-Morán M, Fernández-Vega I, Pérez-Álvarez A, Villafani-Echazú J. Epstein–Barr virus and multiple sclerosis. From evidence to therapeutic strategies. Journal of the Neurological Sciences. 2016;**361**:213-219

[13] Westerlind H, Stawiarz L, Fink K, Hillert J, Manouchehrinia A. A significant decrease in diagnosis of primary progressive multiple sclerosis: A cohort study. Multiple Sclerosis Journal. 2016;**22**(8):1071-1079

[14] Elliott C, Belachew S, Wolinsky JS, Hauser SL, Kappos L, Barkhof F, et al. Chronic white matter lesion activity predicts clinical progression in primary progressive multiple sclerosis. Brain. 2019;**142**(9):2787-2799

[15] Campbell G, Mahad DJ. Mitochondrial dysfunction and axon degeneration in progressive multiple sclerosis. FEBS Letters. 2018;**592**(7):1113-1121

[16] Brownlee WJ, Solanky B, Prados F, Yiannakas M, Da Mota P, Riemer F, et al. Cortical grey matter sodium accumulation is associated with disability and secondary progressive disease course in relapse-onset multiple

sclerosis. Journal of Neurology, Neurosurgery, and Psychiatry. 2019;**90**(7):755-760

[17] Rommer PS, Eichstädt K, Ellenberger D, Flachenecker P, Friede T, Haas J, et al. Symptomatology and symptomatic treatment in multiple sclerosis: Results from a nationwide MS registry. Multiple Sclerosis Journal. 2019;**25**(12):1641-1652

[18] Eijlers AJ, van Geest Q, Dekker I, Steenwijk MD, Meijer KA, Hulst HE, et al. Predicting cognitive decline in multiple sclerosis: A 5-year follow-up study. Brain. 2018;**141**(9):2605-2618

[19] Cabeça HL, Rocha LC, Sabbá AF, Tomás AM, Bento-Torres NV, Anthony DC, et al. The subtleties of cognitive decline in multiple sclerosis: An exploratory study using hierarchical cluster analysis of CANTAB results. BMC Neurology. 2018;**18**(1):140

[20] Sumowski JF, Benedict R, Enzinger C, Filippi M, Geurts JJ, Hamalainen P, et al. Cognition in multiple sclerosis: State of the field and priorities for the future. Neurology. 2018;**90**(6):278-288

[21] Kalatha T, Arnaoutoglou M, Koukoulidis T, Hatzifilippou E, Bouras E, Baloyannis S, et al. Does cognitive dysfunction correlate with neurofilament light polypeptide levels in the CSF of patients with multiple sclerosis? Journal of International Medical Research. 2019;**47**(5):2187-2198

[22] Prouskas SE, Chiaravalloti ND, Kant N, Ball KK, de Groot V, Uitdehaag BM, et al. Cognitive rehabilitation in patients with advanced progressive multiple sclerosis: Possible within limits? Multiple Sclerosis Journal. 2019;**10**:228

[23] Kalatha T, Balogiannis S, Kalathas T, Arnaoutoglou M, Bouras E, Koukoulidis T, et al. The Correlation Between Cognitive Disorders and Clinical Parameters in a Cohort of Greek Multiple Sclerosis Patients. Aristotle University of Thessaloniki; 2018

[24] Renauld S, Mohamed-Said L, Macoir J. Language disorders in multiple sclerosis: A systematic review. Multiple Sclerosis and Related Disorders. 2016;**10**:103-111

[25] Vizza P, Mirarchi D, Tradigo G, Redavide M, Bossio RB, Veltri P. Vocal signal analysis in patients affected by multiple sclerosis. Procedia Computer Science. 2017;**108**:1205-1214

[26] Thompson AJ, Banwell BL, Barkhof F, Carroll WM, Coetzee T, Comi G, et al. Diagnosis of multiple sclerosis: 2017 revisions of the McDonald criteria. The Lancet Neurology. 2018;**17**(2):162-173

[27] Filippi M, Rocca MA, Ciccarelli O, De Stefano N, Evangelou N, Kappos L, et al. MRI criteria for the diagnosis of multiple sclerosis: MAGNIMS consensus guidelines. The Lancet Neurology. 2016;**15**(3):292-303

[28] Knier B, Leppenetier G, Wetzlmair C, Aly L, Hoshi MM, Pernpeintner V, et al. Association of retinal architecture, intrathecal immunity, and clinical course in multiple sclerosis. JAMA Neurology. 2017;**74**(7):847-856

[29] Preziosa P, Rocca MA, Mesaros S, Meani A, Montalban X, Drulovic J, et al. Diagnosis of multiple sclerosis: A multicentre study to compare revised McDonald-2010 and Filippi-2010 criteria. Journal of Neurology, Neurosurgery, and Psychiatry. 2018;**89**(3):316-318

[30] Solomon AJ, Naismith RT, Cross AH. Misdiagnosis of multiple sclerosis: Impact of the 2017 McDonald criteria on clinical practice. Neurology. 2019;**92**(1):26-33

[31] Arrambide G, Tintore M, Espejo C, Auger C, Castillo M, Río J, et al. The value of oligoclonal bands in the multiple sclerosis diagnostic criteria. Brain. 2018;**141**(4):1075-1084

[32] Becker J, Geffken M, Diehl RR, Berlit P, Krämer M. Choosing wisely? Multiple sclerosis and laboratory screening for autoimmune differential diagnoses. Neurology International Open. 2017;**1**(04):E256-E263

[33] Yeshokumar AK, Banwell BL. Diagnostic challenges in pediatric multiple sclerosis and neuromyelitis optica spectrum disorder. Journal of Pediatric Neurology. 2018;**16**(03):185-191

[34] Braz L, Sampaio M, Guimarães J, Leão M. Multiphasic ADEM reclassified in multiple sclerosis: A case with therapeutic implications

[35] López-Chiriboga AS, Majed M, Fryer J, Dubey D, McKeon A, Flanagan EP, et al. Association of MOG-IgG serostatus with relapse after acute disseminated encephalomyelitis and proposed diagnostic criteria for MOG-IgG-associated disorders. JAMA Neurology. 2018;**75**(11):1355-1363

[36] Shahbeigi S, Karamolahi S, Pakdaman H, Nazarbaghi S, Altintas A. The neurological manifestations as an onset symptom of antiphospholipid syndrome: Report of two cases. International Journal of Neurology and Brain Disorders. 2019;**6**(1):1-3

[37] Kleffner I, Dörr J, Ringelstein M, Gross CC, Böckenfeld Y, Schwindt W, et al. Diagnostic criteria for Susac syndrome. Journal of Neurology, Neurosurgery, and Psychiatry. 2016;**87**(12):1287-1295

[38] Matta AP, Nascimento OJ, Ferreira AC, Magalhães TN, Benevides TP, Kirmse A, et al. No evidence of disease activity in multiple sclerosis patients. Expert Review of Neurotherapeutics. 2016;**16**(11):1279-1284

[39] Kappos L, De Stefano N, Freedman MS, Cree BA, Radue EW, Sprenger T, et al. Inclusion of brain volume loss in a revised measure of no evidence of disease activity'(NEDA-4) in relapsing–remitting multiple sclerosis. Multiple Sclerosis Journal. 2016;**22**(10):1297-1305

[40] Comi G, Radaelli M, Sørensen PS. Evolving concepts in the treatment of relapsing multiple sclerosis. The Lancet. 2017;**389**(10076):1347-1356

[41] de Dios López A, Montaña SJ, Parada LS, Broseta PL, Marqués MM, Subirada MC. CP-204 observational study on the use of different therapeutic alternatives for multiple sclerosis treatment

[42] Vidal-Jordana A, Sastre-Garriga J, Rovira A, Montalban X. Treating relapsing–remitting multiple sclerosis: Therapy effects on brain atrophy. Journal of Neurology. 2015;**262**(12):2617-2626

[43] Kalincik T, Manouchehrinia A, Sobisek L, Jokubaitis V, Spelman T, Horakova D, et al. Towards personalized therapy for multiple sclerosis: Prediction of individual treatment response. Brain. 2017;**140**(9):2426-2443

[44] Lublin F. History of modern multiple sclerosis therapy. Journal of Neurology. 2005;**252**(3):iii3-iii9

[45] Karni A, Abraham M, Monsonego A, Cai G, Freeman GJ, Hafler D, et al. Innate immunity in multiple sclerosis: Myeloid dendritic cells in secondary progressive multiple sclerosis are activated and drive a proinflammatory immune response. The Journal of Immunology. 2006;**177**(6):4196-4202

[46] Mishra MK, Yong VW. Myeloid cells—Targets of medication in multiple sclerosis. Nature Reviews. Neurology. 2016;**12**(9):539-551

[47] Hemmer B, Kerschensteiner M, Korn T. Role of the innate and adaptive immune responses in the course of multiple sclerosis. The Lancet Neurology. 2015;**14**(4):406-419

[48] Pender MP, Csurhes PA, Smith C, Beagley L, Hooper KD, Raj M, et al. Epstein–Barr virus-specific adoptive immunotherapy for progressive multiple sclerosis. Multiple Sclerosis Journal. 2014;**20**(11):1541-1544

[49] Patti F. Optimizing the benefit of multiple sclerosis therapy: The importance of treatment adherence. Patient Preference and Adherence. 2010;**4**:1

[50] Kesselring J, Beer S. Symptomatic therapy and neurorehabilitation in multiple sclerosis. The Lancet Neurology. 2005;**4**(10):643-652

[51] Yadav V, Marracci G, Kim E, Spain R, Cameron M, Overs S, et al. Low-fat, plant-based diet in multiple sclerosis: A randomized controlled trial. Multiple Sclerosis and Related Disorders. 2016;**9**:80-90

[52] White LJ, Castellano V. Exercise and brain health—Implications for multiple sclerosis. Sports Medicine. 2008;**38**(2):91-100

[53] MacAllister WS, Krupp LB. Multiple sclerosis-related fatigue. Physical Medicine and Rehabilitation Clinics of North America. 2005;**16**(2):483-502

[54] Taylor P, Dorstyn DS, Prior E. Stress management interventions for multiple sclerosis: A meta-analysis of randomized controlled trials. Journal of Health Psychology. 2019:1359105319860185

[55] Navidi-Moghadam M, Saffarinia M, Alipour A, Sahraian MA. Comparison of the effectiveness of mindfulness-based-cognitive-therapy and solution-focused group therapy on the perception of social support and interpersonal relationships among patients with multiple sclerosis. Salamat Ijtimai (Community Health). 2019;**6**(3):342-356

[56] Schmid W, Aldridge D. Active music therapy in the treatment of multiple sclerosis patients: A matched control study. Journal of Music Therapy. 2004;**41**(3):225-240

[57] LeDoux J, Mann C, Demoratz M, Young J. Addressing spiritual and religious influences in care delivery. Professional Case Management. 2019;**24**(3):142-147

Section 2

Etiopathology

Chapter 2

Myeloid Cells in Multiple Sclerosis

Marilyn Wang, Sofia Caryotakis, Nagendra Kumar Rai, Alan Nguyen and Athena M. Soulika

Abstract

In steady state, the central nervous system (CNS) houses a variety of myeloid cells, such as microglia, non-parenchymal macrophages and dendritic cells (DCs), and granulocytes. Most of these cells enter the CNS during embryogenesis and are crucial for proper CNS development. In adulthood, these resident myeloid cells exert crucial homeostatic functions. In neuroinflammatory conditions, like multiple sclerosis (MS), both lymphoid and myeloid cells from the periphery infiltrate the tissue and cause local damage. Although lymphocytes are undeniably important players in MS, CNS-resident and CNS-infiltrating myeloid cells have recently gained much-deserved attention for their roles in disease progression. Here, we will review significant advances made in recent years delineating myeloid cell functions within the CNS both in homeostasis and MS. We will also discuss how these cells are affected by currently employed therapeutics for MS patients.

Keywords: microglia, macrophages, dendritic cells, monocytes, granulocytes, disease modifying treatments, multiple sclerosis, EAE

1. Introduction

Myeloid cells are crucial for central nervous system (CNS) tissue function both in development and adulthood. Other than microglia, which are found in the parenchyma, CNS meningeal and perivascular spaces along with the choroid plexus, are populated by special subsets of macrophages and dendritic cells [1–3]. Additionally, granulocyte cells are also present in the homeostatic CNS [4]. Studies in rodents have elucidated mechanisms by which these cells promote tissue physiology.

In multiple sclerosis (MS), myeloid cells play a dominant role. Studies in mice and human patient samples show that myeloid cells from the periphery enter the tissue through a compromised blood-brain barrier (BBB) and together with CNS-resident cells perpetuate the inflammatory environment through secretion of inflammatory cytokines and reactivation of primed T cells. However, myeloid cells may also exhibit anti-inflammatory and pro-reparative functions. The exact contribution of each myeloid subset to disease progression is currently the focus of thorough investigation.

Here, we will provide an overview of myeloid cell types and functions in homeostasis and how these populations evolve in neuroinflammation. In addition, we will review the effects of therapeutics currently employed for MS patients on myeloid cell populations and functions.

2. CNS-resident myeloid cells in homeostasis

The CNS houses a variety of myeloid cell subsets that exert multiple functions crucial to homeostasis such as BBB maintenance, sampling of the local milieu, synaptic pruning, and control of neuronal populations in development and adulthood. In this section, we will elaborate on the developmental origin and known functions of these subsets in the CNS.

2.1 Microglia

Microglia are resident immune cells within the CNS parenchyma proper. They derive from Runx1+ erythromyeloid precursors in the extraembryonic yolk sac and enter the brain early in embryonic development [5–7]. Before migrating out of the yolk sac, these progenitors acquire CD45 and CX3CR1 expression [8] and seed the brain parenchyma around embryonic day 9.5 [7, 9, 10], through a process that is mediated largely by the metalloproteinases MMP8 and MMP9 [8].

Microglia development relies on transcription factors PU.1, IRF8, and colony-stimulating factor 1 receptor (CSF1R) signaling [11], whereas transcription factors such as MYB, BATF3, and ID2 are not necessary, suggesting that microglia are transcriptionally distinct from bone marrow-derived myeloid cells [6, 10]. Moreover, the microglial transcriptional profile changes at each developmental stage, roughly divided into early microglia (microglia that seed the brain from E10.5 to E12.5), pre-microglia (microglia found in the CNS from E12.5 up to P9), and adult microglia [10, 12]. Early microglia are highly proliferative, pre-microglia exert functions on synapse pruning [10] and excess neuron elimination [13], and adult microglia perform immune surveillance but also synaptic refinement [11, 14–16]. During development, microglia control the numbers of neural progenitors via phagocytosis. This was shown by clodronate-mediated microglia deletion in organotypic brain cultures [13] or in CSF1R knockout mice, which lack microglia [17]. However, CSF1R is also expressed in other cells including peripheral myeloid subsets and neurons. Specific deletion of CSF1R in nestin+ cells recapitulated some of the observed effects in the global CSF1R knockout [17].

Complement components C1q and C3 tag extra synapses which are then removed by microglia via CR3 receptor-mediated phagocytosis [15, 16]. This process is known as synaptic pruning [15]. Neuronally derived CX3CL1 acting on microglial CX3CR1 is one of the cues that guide microglia to the synapses [15]. Mice deficient in microglia or CX3CR1 exhibit neuronal connectivity and behavioral deficits similar to those observed in autism spectrum disorders [4, 10, 18, 19]. Developing microglia also control neural cells in the cerebellum and were shown to induce Purkinje cell death via NADPH activity [5, 20]. On the other hand, developing microglia also secrete trophic factors that promote neuronal circuit formation and neuronal survival. Microglial-derived insulin-like growth factor 1 (IGF-1) promotes survival of cortical layer V neurons in postnatal development. In addition, it induces the fate of many cell lineages, such as oligodendrocytes, and also protects them from glutamate-mediated apoptosis [5]. Basic fibroblast growth factor, hepatocyte growth factor, epidermal growth factor, platelet-derived growth factor, nerve growth factor, and brain-derived neurotrophic factor are all also secreted by microglia and contribute to neuronal development, maintenance, and function throughout life [21–23].

As microglia mature, they adopt a ramified morphology characterized by a small body and thin, long processes. Interestingly, recent studies suggest that adult microglia are not a homogeneous population and their activation state is the result of region-specific cues [24–30]. They are self-renewing via a local progenitor [31, 32], but in certain instances and when microglia are depleted for prolonged periods of time via genetic or pharmacologic methods, peripheral myeloid cells can enter and engraft in the CNS for long periods but remain functionally distinct [33]. Microglia in the steady-state CNS depend on CSF1R signaling for survival. Both CSF1R ligands, CSF1 and IL-34, are found in the normal CNS and their expression is regionally controlled [34]. Interestingly, in the absence of CSF1, microglia numbers decrease by 30%, while in the absence of IL-34, microglial numbers decrease by 70%. IL-34 in particular controls the migration of microglial precursor cells in the CNS via CSF1R signaling in development [35]. TGF-β signaling is also necessary for homeostatic microglial functions, and in its absence, they assume a transcriptome that is similar to that of peripheral macrophages [36].

Defining microglial markers that are distinct from those of peripheral monocytes has been the focus of investigation for many years. New RNA-Seq techniques yielded a number of genes that are preferentially expressed by microglia but not peripheral myeloid cells in homeostasis [1, 10, 18, 37, 38]. Lately, the most commonly employed markers are the purinergic receptor P2Y, G-protein coupled receptor 12 (P2RY12), the transmembrane protein TMEM119, and the transcriptional regulator Sal-like 1 (SALL1) [1, 10, 18, 37, 38]. Both P2RY12 and TMEM119 are expressed by the vast majority of microglia within the healthy CNS. The function of TMEM119 in microglia has not been yet elucidated, but in other cell types, it has been implicated with differentiation and proliferation [39–42]. P2RY12 serves as a chemotactic receptor that guides microglia to sites of injury [26]. SALL1 is a microglia fate-determining factor, vital for expression of essential microglial genes and normal microglial morphology [26, 36]. Whether these markers are still able to differentiate between microglia and infiltrating myeloid cells in neuroinflammation, when all these cells undergo major transcriptional changes, is still under investigation. However, SALL1 and TMEM119 are emerging as the most reliable microglial markers.

Adult microglia exert multiple roles in tissue maintenance: they phagocytose debris or dead cells, clear toxic amyloid-β, shape neural circuits via phagocytosing inappropriate or inactive connections [16], provide trophic support to neurons by producing growth factors, and regulate neurogenesis in the hippocampus and the subventricular zone (SVZ). Interestingly, microglial-derived CX3CL1 increases with exercise and confers a protective effect on neuronal cells, while CX3CR1 deletion results in activated microglia with an inflammatory phenotype, leading to decreased rates of adult neurogenesis in the hippocampus [43–45]. In addition, microglia phagocytose neuronal progenitors in the adult SVZ, thus controlling the local pool of neurons [18, 44, 46]. Microglia also influence oligodendrocyte development and myelinogenesis both during development and in adulthood. In the adult CNS, microglia are necessary for myelin homeostasis and maintenance of adult oligodendrocyte progenitor cells [47, 48], promote BBB function [49, 50], and in case of injury, they migrate to the affected site to promote repair [51].

Microglial malfunction is associated with neurodegenerative diseases such as Alzheimer's disease, Parkinson's disease, and neurodevelopmental and psychological defects such as Rett syndrome and obsessive-compulsive disorder [10]. Furthermore, the lack of phagocytosis by microglia results in excess synapses which is associated with impaired memory formation [16].

2.2 Tissue-resident macrophages

In addition to microglia, the healthy CNS houses three types of non-parenchymal tissue-resident macrophages. They are named based on their location and are currently categorized as perivascular macrophages, meningeal macrophages, and macrophages in the choroid plexus [1, 52]. These macrophage populations are optimally placed to regulate and interrogate peripheral cell entry, act as sentinels by sampling their environment, and quickly respond in the event of an insult. Previously thought to be derived from bone marrow (BM) monocytic progenitor cells, it is now established that the majority of CNS-resident macrophages are long-lived and transcriptionally similar to microglia. As such, most of these cells are derived from erythromyeloid progenitors found in the extraembryonic yolk sac or the fetal liver, and their generation is dependent on PU.1 and independent of MYB and BATF3 [1, 7]. Choroid plexus macrophages are the most distinct among these types of CNS non-parenchymal macrophages and originate from either embryonic precursors or BM.

Perivascular macrophages are located between the blood vessel endothelium (of BBB) and the glia limitans, which form the barrier for the CNS parenchyma. They are wrapped around endothelial walls with their elongated cell bodies and monitor the perivascular space [2]. Perivascular macrophages provide nutrients to endothelial cells, regulate vascular permeability, maintain BBB integrity, clear toxic amyloid-β from the CNS, sample debris to assess the local milieu, and communicate with surrounding cells [52]. Their location is ideal to simultaneously sample both the CNS interstitial fluid and the blood [1, 52]. Perivascular macrophages infiltrate the CNS at the same time as microglia (E 9.5) and populate the abluminal spaces of the newly developed vasculature. Together with microglia, these macrophages play significant roles on the refinements of the developing vasculature [53]. In adulthood and in response to injury, perivascular macrophages promote anastomoses and the repair of vasculature [54].

Meningeal macrophages have a very similar origin and transcriptional control as perivascular macrophages. They are located in between meningeal vasculature and ER-TR7+ fibroblast-like cells that line the meninges. They also express similar markers to those of perivascular macrophages and are also long-lived with negligible contribution from the periphery [1, 2].

The choroid plexus macrophages reside on the apical side of the epithelium facing the cerebrospinal fluid (CSF) in the stroma. The stroma of the choroid plexus is highly vascularized and surrounded by a monolayer of cuboidal epithelial cells, which are joined together by tight junctions forming the blood-CSF barrier. The choroid plexus is located in all four ventricles of the brain and is responsible for producing CSF [52]. It allows trafficking of a variety of immune cell types and is an area with an anti-inflammatory environment [55, 56]. In addition, the choroid plexus is the gateway to the CNS and is an area through which pioneering T cells gain access into the CNS in preclinical stages of the MS murine model experimental autoimmune encephalomyelitis (EAE) [57]. Unlike the other types of CNS macrophages, these macrophages are partially replenished from the bone marrow [1].

All of these brain-resident macrophages express the mannose receptor CD206 and scavenger receptor CD163, along with CD11b, CX3CR1, and MHC-II. Perivascular and meningeal macrophages also express the lymphatic vessel endothelial hyaluronan receptor LYVE1, which is not expressed in choroid plexus-associated macrophages [1, 2, 58].

2.3 Dendritic cells

At steady state, dendritic cells (DCs) are sparsely distributed within the non-parenchymal CNS spaces. They are more numerous in the leptomeninges and dura mater, less prominent in the choroid plexus, and mostly absent from perivascular spaces [3].

DCs develop from committed DC or monocyte progenitors in the BM and are dependent upon FLT3 signaling [59]. They are relatively short-lived and are replenished roughly every 1–2 weeks [60]. Mature DCs are divided into conventional DCs (cDCs), plasmacytoid DCs (pDCs), and monocyte-derived DCs (moDCs). cDCs are further subdivided into cDC1 and cDC2. cDC1s are associated with Th1 responses [61, 62], while cDC2 with Th2 and Th17 [63]. cDC1s are also able to cross present antigens and activate CD8+ T cells. cDCs leave the BM in the form of committed precursors, while pDCs mature in the BM before entering the circulation. In addition, moDCs are not usually found in steady state but are crucial mediators on inflammatory responses [64].

IRF4 and IRF8 are transcription factors differentially expressed in the various DC subsets. cDC1s are IRF8+IRF4lo/−, cDC2s are IRF8loIRF4+, pDCs are IRF8+IRF4+, and moDCs are IRF4loIRF8lo [65]. cDC1s do not express CD11b. Within the mouse CNS, the majority of DCs are cDC2 and are mostly located in the leptomeninges and dura mater, while in the choroid plexus, the majority of DCs are cDC1s [3].

2.4 Granulocytes

Although their presence within the CNS at steady state is commonly ignored, various types of granulocytes such as neutrophils, mast cells, basophils, and eosinophils are found within perivascular and meningeal spaces and the choroid plexus [4]. Mast cells in particular are also found within the parenchyma [66, 67].

Neutrophils exit the bone marrow in a mature state and are thought to be short-lived. However, subsets of neutrophils live much longer than previously thought and, more importantly, some have been found in various organs likely as a local reservoir [68]. It is now acknowledged that neutrophils or neutrophil subsets may have different functions. Other than the well-documented inflammatory functions, pro-reparative CD206+ neutrophils, VEGF-responding angiogenic neutrophils, and CD11c+Ly6G+ “hybrid” cell types have been identified [69–72]. Interestingly, neutrophils were recently detected in the normal murine CNS localized within the subdural meningeal spaces, but their contribution to tissue homeostasis is still not known [73].

Mast cells (MCs) are derived from CD34+ bone marrow progenitor cells, enter the circulation in an immature state, and mature once they reach the tissue in response to local cues. They are mostly known for their effects during allergic/atopic responses mediated by cross-linking of their FcεRI receptor by IgE. MCs are a heterogeneous population, and depending on the types of proteases they carry within their granules, they are broadly categorized into at least three subtypes: MCs that contain only tryptase (MCT), MCs that contain only chymase (MCC), and MCs that contain tryptase, chymase, carboxypeptidase, and cathepsin G (MCCT) [74, 75]. MCs are loaded with granules containing preformed mediators and can synthesize mediators de novo. They are found in many tissues and usually associated with vascular epithelial cells and nerves. CNS MCs are constitutively active and degranulate in response to homeostatic or inflammatory stimuli [67, 76–78]. Their preformed granules are released immediately upon activation and contain various mediators such as histamine, serotonin, and TNF-α in addition to proteases. They can quickly synthesize lipid mediators such as prostaglandins and leukotrienes and growth factors. A late-phase MC activation results in de novo production of inflammatory cytokines such as IL-6 and TNF-α [74, 79].

Within the healthy CNS, MCs are found within the thalamus, hypothalamus, entorhinal cortex, hippocampus, meninges, and perivascular spaces in proximity to the BBB. They interact with neurons and microglia, and their granules contain a plethora of mediators including neurotransmitters. Their location allows them to modulate BBB permeability, and genetically modified mice that lack MCs display decreased BBB permeability both in homeostasis and neuroinflammation [67, 77, 78].

MC activity in stress has been associated with migraines [78, 80]. Moreover, histamine released from MCs was shown to promote wakefulness in adult mice [81] and microglial synaptic pruning in the developing CNS, which then regulates sexual behavior in adulthood [82].

3. Myeloid cells in multiple sclerosis

Pathologically, MS is characterized by focal demyelinating lesions disseminated in space and time and neuronal and axonal damage. MS lesions are rich in myeloid cells (microglia, infiltrating monocyte-derived macrophages, and DCs), which outnumber lymphoid cells [83]. Below we will discuss current knowledge on myeloid cells in MS, which are now emerging as crucial players in disease pathogenesis and progression. Some of this knowledge is derived from studies on the animal model of MS, experimental autoimmune encephalomyelitis (EAE). Although this model has been criticized [84], it mimics most of the CNS pathology observed in MS such as tissue infiltration by immune cells, formation of lesions, local inflammation, and progressive axonal loss [85, 86].

Monocytes are not found in the healthy CNS but are regularly found in the CNS and CSF of MS patients. Once they enter the CNS, monocytes mature into macrophages and participate in disease progression. There are three well-characterized monocyte subsets categorized based on expression patterns of the LPS receptor CD14 and the Fce (greek) RIII receptor CD16: the classical CD14++CD16- (similar to the inflammatory monocyte Ly6ChiCCR2+ in mice), the nonclassical CD14+CD16++ (similar to the anti-inflammatory CX3CR1+Ly6Clo in mice), and the intermediate CD14++CD16+. CD16+ monocytes have been associated with inflammation and promoting the generation of Th17 cells. MS patients with active disease show increased CD14+ cells both in the blood and the CSF. These cells also contribute to BBB disruption [87, 88].

Both conventional and plasmacytoid DCs are increased in the blood and CSF of MS patients. cDCs are usually found early in disease, and pDC numbers are highly increased in the CSF during relapses. Circulating cDCs in MS patients upregulate CCR5 which is a receptor for CCL3 and CCL5, both of which are upregulated in MS lesions. However, cDCs in primary progressive MS display an immature phenotype [89]. Interestingly, although pDC numbers increase in MS, these cells are found to be phenotypically similar to those of healthy controls. Although the data on circulating pDCs are still conflicting, imbalances in DC populations may result in significant changes in T-cell functionally in MS [90].

3.1 Myeloid cells in MS lesions

MS lesions are found both within the brain and spinal cord and can be formed within the white and the gray matter [91, 92]. The most commonly employed classification is the four types of lesions described by Lucchinetti and colleagues [93]. Type I is characterized by macrophage products, and type II is characterized by antibody and complement deposition, while type III lacks complement and antibody deposition. Types I and II have clearly demarcated borders, while type III is characterized by diffuse demyelination and lacks clear demarcation. Type IV is characterized by dystrophic apoptotic oligodendrocytes. In most of these lesions, the major cell types are myeloid cells [83].

Although more pronounced during relapses, infiltrating myeloid cells and activated microglia are found within the CNS of MS patients throughout the disease and are associated with demyelination, oligodendrocytic loss, and axonal damage [92, 94, 95]. With the exception of rapid progressive MS, in which the CNS is intensely infiltrated [94], in progressive forms of the disease, the tissue is not massively infiltrated; however, myeloid cells (microglia and/or infiltrating myeloid) remain activated [92, 96]. During progressive stages of the disease, axonal loss is prominent leading to tissue atrophy in both MS and EAE [86, 92]. These processes are likely mediated via the production of oxygen radicals produced by either microglia or infiltrating myeloid cells [84].

3.1.1 Microglia/macrophages

The contribution of microglia to MS is still debated. Studies in mice have shown that microglia are poor antigen-presenting cells and not likely to activate infiltrating lymphocytes. Instead, microglia may contribute to the disease process via oxidative stress and production of pro-inflammatory cytokines that may activate astrocytes or cause oligodendrocytic damage. Microglia are highly phagocytic and thus can remove myelin debris and cellular fragments, damaged axons, and dead cells. It is clear that microglia are activated in the CNS of MS patients, but whether they promote disease or facilitate repair is still not well delineated. One of the main hurdles for these investigations is that there is no unique marker to reliably distinguish microglia from infiltrating monocytes in neuroinflammation. Additionally, activated microglia are morphologically indistinguishable from infiltrating monocytes/macrophages. RNA transcriptome analysis has yielded a number of markers that show preferential expression in microglia (see Section 2.1). TMEM119 is the only marker so far examined in MS tissue and seems to be expressed by a subpopulation of myeloid cells within lesions and in cells with microglial morphology in nonlesional areas [97]. However, there is still not a wide breadth of studies examining the specificity of TMEM119 in neuroinflammation, when all myeloid cells undergo major transcriptional changes [2]. Thus, below we will talk about microglia and macrophages as one population in active MS lesions and specify TMEM119-expressing cells within the MS CNS.

Microglia/macrophages (M/Ms) in active MS lesions are heterogeneous and capable of performing a variety of activities that may promote or control inflammation and repair [98, 99]. M/Ms found within active MS lesions usually express markers associated with inflammatory macrophage functions, including inducible nitric oxide synthase (iNOS), co-stimulatory molecules CD40 and CD86, the Fc receptors CD32 and CD64, phagocytosis marker CD68, and p22phox, a subunit of NADPH oxidase [100, 101]. In addition, M/Ms may also express anti-inflammatory markers such as the mannose receptor CD206 and the scavenger receptor CD163 [100]. Approximately half of the myeloid cells within active lesions express TMEM119, suggesting these cells may be microglia. Interestingly, PY2R12, which is usually expressed in homeostatic microglia, is not expressed in these cells, suggesting it is downregulated upon activation [97].

MS lesions are not static and over time grow outward, eventually becoming chronically active. These lesions are slowly expanding and have a thin border of M/Ms. The center of these lesions appears quiescent and populated by lipid-laden (foamy) macrophages, many of them expressing CD206 and CD163 [98, 102]. However, M/Ms lining the rim of these lesions express iNOS and HLA-DR, suggesting they are inflammatory and promote T-cell functions [103]. M/Ms at the rims of either active or chronically active plaques contain iron which has been suggested to promote MS pathology [104, 105]. In the normal CNS, most iron is found within oligodendrocytes or myelin. When iron is released after oligodendrocytic death and demyelination, it is internalized by ferritin+ M/Ms which acquire a dystrophic phenotype [106]. Interestingly TMEM119+ cells that express low or no P2RY12 (likely activated microglia) are found within chronically active or slow-expanding lesions, and their density decreases inward. Strikingly, there are no differences between overall M/M density and levels of activation between lesion types [97, 100, 103].

Areas of the CNS that are far from the demyelinating lesions and often appearing normal (normal-appearing white matter; NAWM) are also characterized by scattered microglial activation. Interestingly, ramified microglia were shown to express iNOS and were often close to injured axons [107]. However, microglia have also been documented to exhibit a suppressed and anti-inflammatory character [108]. Clusters of microglia or macrophages, known as microglial nodules, have been found in NAWM in close proximity to degenerating axons. These nodules appear in the absence of extensive inflammation, astrogliosis, or demyelination, and their formation has been argued to be one of the early events in MS pathology [109]. Furthermore, P2RY12+ TMEM119+ microglia in the NAWM also expressing activation markers CD68 and p22phox are found in both MS and healthy controls' brains, suggesting that certain microglial populations are in a pre-activated state [97].

In addition to white matter, demyelination is also observed within the gray matter. MS gray matter is characterized by less infiltration by immune cells and less activation of M/Ms compared to white matter. This type of demyelination has been mostly attributed to aberrant microglia functions such as ROS production via the NADPH oxidase activity. This mechanism seems to be more prominent in the gray matter compared to white matter lesions. In addition, cortical microglial activation can be observed via PET imaging by administering the traditional PK11195 and more recently the novel PBR28 ligand [110, 111].

In progressive forms of MS, M/Ms are activated both within the lesions and in the normal-appearing white and gray matter, and this has been linked to inflammatory cytokines produced in the meninges, likely by infiltrating B cells [112, 113]. Activated complement component 3 fragments (C3d) are found within microglia clusters of slowly expanding lesions in progressive but not acute MS [114] and in close proximity of damaged axons. This suggests that C3 activation and deposition are not likely associated with lesion initiation but rather a mechanism that facilitates the removal of axonal and cellular debris. Furthermore, the activation/phagocytosis marker CD68 is significantly increased in the NAWM in progressive forms of MS compared to that of relapsing–remitting MS and healthy controls [97].

3.1.2 Dendritic cells

Both cDCs and pDCs accumulate in the leptomeninges and lesions in MS patients. MoDCs, which are not present in the homeostatic CNS, differentiate from infiltrating inflammatory monocytes after these reach the CNS of MS patients. Studies in murine EAE showed that both cDCs and moDCs are found within the CNS infiltrates. cDCs express CD26 and ZBTB46, a transcription factor also expressed in human cDCs, while moDCs express CD88 and CD64 [3, 103, 115]. Although these markers may be expressed by other cell types, they are useful markers for identification of DC subsets. cDCs are the most efficient antigen-presenting cells and are able to process larger myelin fragments to activate naive and effector T cells. Both cDCs and moDCs progressively expand during the onset and peak of EAE in every CNS compartment. pDCs are not efficient antigen-presenting cells but are equipped to secrete inflammatory cytokines and promote an inflammatory environment to support cDCs and moDCs [116].

3.1.3 Granulocytes

Neutrophils are relatively rare in established MS lesions; thus, their contribution to disease course has long been debated. Studies in EAE show that neutrophils are part of the inflammatory lesions, appear early in disease process [86, 117], and are increased in peripheral lymphoid organs and blood [117]. Neutrophils may promote early disease progression by increasing permeability of the BBB, possibly through secretion of matrix metalloproteinases or the release of neutrophil extracellular traps (NETs) [118, 119]. Inactivation of neutrophil products, such as myeloperoxidase or neutrophil elastase, results in milder EAE course and associated optic neuritis [120, 121]. In agreement with the EAE data, CSF of newly diagnosed patients shows elevated neutrophil counts [122], and the CSF of patients with established disease contains increased levels of the neutrophil chemoattractant CXCL8 [123, 124]. Neutrophil elastase and chemokines that promote neutrophil recruitment, such as CXCL1 and CXCL5, are systemically elevated in relapsing MS patients and correlate with lesion burden and clinical disability [125]. Transcripts of the granulocyte colony-stimulating factor (G-CSF) which promotes the proliferation and differentiation of neutrophils (and other granulocytes) are found within lesions but not in NAWM [126], and treatment with G-CSF worsens MS symptoms [127, 128]. Thus, lack of neutrophil detection in MS lesions may be due to incorrect sampling timing.

Interestingly, mast cells are found in close proximity to MS lesions and were initially observed in 1890 by Neuman [129] and later by other groups [66, 130–132]. Their numbers are very low compared with those of the other myeloid subsets; thus, not much is known about their contribution to disease progression. However, the ability of mast cells to secrete histamine and proteases may facilitate disease onset or relapses by promoting vascular permeability and tissue infiltration. In EAE, mice with spontaneous c-Kit mutations that lead to deletion of mast cells have shown that these cells may prevent, promote, or have no effect on disease onset and progression [133]. These conflicting data are likely due to the fact that none of these mouse strains are specific and efficient mast cell knockouts.

4. Effect of MS therapeutics on myeloid cells

MS therapies are designed to dampen immune system activation. Although most of these therapies target lymphocytes, myeloid cells can also be affected directly or indirectly. This section will explore how current MS therapies affect myeloid cells.

4.1 IFN-β

IFN-β, the first FDA-approved biologic therapeutic for MS, is a pleiotropic cytokine exerting a plethora of effects on a variety of cells [134, 135]. Monocytes isolated from MS patients treated ex vivo with IFN-β exhibit impaired inflammatory responses when stimulated with LPS/alum compared to monocytes isolated from healthy donors [136]. Ex vivo treatment of DCs derived from MS patients or healthy donors with IFN-β reduced the expression of IL-1β and IL-23 and upregulated the expression of IL-12p35 and IL-27p28, which resulted in reduced generation of Th17 cells [137]. Additionally, studies in EAE showed that deletion of IFN-α/β receptor (IFNAR), the receptor of IFN-β specifically on myeloid cells, resulted in aggravated EAE disease [138].

IFN-β is one of the most common first-line MS treatments; however, a large proportion of patients is not responsive. Interestingly, non-responders exhibit exaggerated upregulation of type I IFN-responsive genes either at baseline or in response to IFN-β treatment compared to responders [139–141]. MS patients that upregulated the death-associated receptor TRAIL on monocytes were responsive to IFN-b treatment, but those who did not upregulate TRAIL were not responsive to IFN-b treatment. than patients that did not [142]. Additionally, monocytes isolated from MS patients treated with IFN-β for prolonged periods of time (9 months to 6 years) upregulated the co-stimulatory molecules CD80, CD86, and CD40 [143], and were associated with responsiveness to treatment [144]. A different study, however, showed a positive association between monocytic CD40 upregulation, early after IFN-β injections (9–12 h) and relapses [145].

About 30% of MS patients treated with IFN-β also develop antidrug antibodies and thus are not responsive to treatment. Antidrug antibody generation was associated with decreased NOTCH2 signaling. NOTCH2, which promotes the conversion of patrolling inflammatory monocytes to anti-inflammatory phenotype [146], was markedly reduced in CD14+ monocytes of untreated MS patients that developed antidrug antibodies 12 months after IFN-β therapy initiation [147].

All the above suggest that defining myeloid cell subset propensities in MS before and after treatment initiation will be useful in determining whether IFN-β is a suitable treatment for specific patients.

4.2 Glatiramer acetate

Glatiramer acetate (GA) is a synthetic random copolymer, composed of glutamic acid, alanine, lysine and tyrosine, employed as a treatment for relapsing-remitting MS. MS patients treated with GA show a shift toward Th2 responses and produce anti-inflammatory/pro-repair mediators, likely due to GA effects on myeloid subsets [148, 149]. Initial studies showed that GA binds to MHC-II, altering the myelin antigen presentation capabilities resulting in impaired activation of autoreactive T cells [150, 151]. However, it was later shown that GA can also exert its anti-inflammatory effects independently of MHC-II [152]. Instead, GA was shown to promote the generation of anti-inflammatory monocytes which support regulatory T-cell functions [152].

In support of this, monocytes isolated from the blood of GA-treated MS patients produced significantly higher amounts of IL-10 and lower amounts of IL-12, and the levels of CD16+ anti-inflammatory monocytes were restored to those of healthy controls [153, 154]. DCs from GA-treated MS patients exhibit reduced IL-12 production [155] and express lower levels of CD40, upregulation of which is associated with relapses [156]. Furthermore, the activity of myeloid-derived suppressor cells, a population that suppresses inflammatory responses, is augmented in GA-treated MS patients [157], and GA-treated human microglia express IL-10 and reduce production of pro-inflammatory TNF-α [153]. Increased levels of circulating IL-27, a regulatory cytokine produced by myeloid cells in inflammatory conditions, was recently linked to better GA therapeutic outcomes [158]. Another study showed increased levels of IL-27 in blood, CSF and lesions of MS patients. however, there was no association with treatments [159].

4.3 Fingolimod

Fingolimod is the first oral therapy approved to treat relapsing-remitting MS and is more effective in reducing relapses than IFN-β [160]. Fingolimod (FTY720) is phosphorylated by sphingosine kinase, and its phosphorylated metabolite (FTY720-P) binds to the G-protein-coupled sphingosine-1-phosphate (S1P) receptors. S1P receptors are expressed on a variety of cells including neural, glial, and endothelial cells in the CNS and most of the immune cells in the CNS and the periphery [161]. One of the mechanisms by which fingolimod reduces disease severity and relapses in MS is that it binds S1PR1, a type of S1P receptor, on lymphocytes and prevents their egress from lymphoid tissues [162].

Fingolimod's immunosuppressive effects are also exerted on myeloid cells. Incubation of murine macrophages or human monocytes with either S1P (the natural ligand of S1PR1), or fingolimod, respectively, reduced inflammatory responses after LPS exposure [163–165]. Although microglia, DCs, and peripheral macrophages express similar patterns and levels of S1P receptors, fingolimod downregulated ERK phosphorylation only in DCs and macrophages. Fingolimod also downregulated expression of the pro-inflammatory cytokine IL-12 and upregulated anti-inflammatory IL-10 in DCs and macrophages but not in microglia [164]. Fingolimod crosses the BBB [168], and therapeutic administration of fingolimod reduced TNF-α production by microglia and monocytes in EAE [163]. Flow cytometry analyses of DCs and monocytes isolated from MS patients before and during fingolimod treatment showed decreased levels of activation markers (CD83, CD150, and HLA-DR). Furthermore, fingolimod treatment reduced pro-inflammatory cytokine production, phagocytic activity of DCs and monocytes, and impaired priming of Th1 and Th17 cells [166]. Interestingly, monocytes isolated from fingolimod-treated MS patients exhibited reduced expression of pro-inflammatory micro-RNA miR-155 but also of antioxidant genes HMOX1 and OSGIN1 compared to untreated patients [167]. When monocyte-derived macrophages and microglia were examined in vitro, fingolimod reduced LPS-induced inflammatory cytokines and increased expression of antioxidants. These data suggest that the effects of fingolimod on myeloid cells in vivo may be an indirect effect.

4.4 Dimethyl fumarate

Dimethyl fumarate (DMF) was approved as an oral first-line therapeutic for relapsing-remitting MS in 2013. It is a methyl ester of fumaric acid, quickly metabolized to active monomethyl fumarate which activates transcription factor nuclear factor erythroid-derived 2 (Nrf2) and suppresses NF-κB to modulate oxidative stress [169]. DMF exerts its effects on multiple immune subsets [170].

Monocytes from DMF-treated RRMS patients express reduced levels of the pro-inflammatory micro-RNA miR-155, and DMF-treated human microglia and monocyte-derived macrophages had reduced production of pro-inflammatory cytokines after LPS stimulation, indicating direct regulatory effects [167].

DMF reduces neuroinflammation levels and cognitive deficits induced by systemic LPS administration in mice [171]. In EAE, DMF promoted the generation of anti-inflammatory monocytes and decreased macrophage infiltration into the CNS resulting in milder clinical deficits. Interestingly, these effects were exerted independently of Nrf2 [172, 173].

4.5 Teriflunomide

Teriflunomide is a reversible inhibitor of dihydroorotate dehydrogenase (DHODH), a mitochondrial enzyme active in proliferating cells [174]. Teriflunomide impairs proliferation of lymphocytes, but exerts nebulous effects on myeloid cells [175]. In EAE, teriflunomide reduced T-cell and myeloid cell infiltration of the CNS [176]. In cultured primary microglia, teriflunomide downregulated expression of CD86 and mildly upregulated of IL-10 [177]. Ex vivo, teriflunomide treatment decreased production of IL-6 and CCL2 in activated monocytes from healthy individuals [178].

Furthermore, MS patients after 6 months of treatment showed increased IL-10 production and PD-L1 expression in monocytes, implying that teriflunomide induces anti-inflammatory and regulatory responses in these cells [179].

4.6 Monoclonal antibodies

Several recently developed antibody-based MS therapies target lymphocytes. Below, we will discuss whether and how these therapies affect myeloid cells.

4.6.1 Natalizumab

Natalizumab (NTZ) is an immunomodulatory antibody that limits immune cell infiltration into the CNS by blocking the interaction between the very late activation antigen-4 (VLA-4), an integrin expressed on lymphocytes and myeloid cells, and vascular adhesion molecule-1 (VCAM-1) [180]. As a result, fewer cells are able to migrate and infiltrate the CNS [181]. NTZ reduces relapses and lesion load but increases the risk for progressive multifocal leukoencephalopathy [182]. NTZ reduced the frequencies of mature activated pDCs; however, this activation was not a direct effect of NTZ on pDCs [183].

Triggering receptor 2 expressed on myeloid cells (TREM2) is an innate immune receptor associated with inflammatory responses and within the CNS expressed by microglia [184]. In neuroinflammation, microglia shed TREM2, which can be detected in CSF [185, 186]. NTZ reduced CSF-soluble TREM2 to baseline levels, indicating dampened microglial activation, which is associated with improved clinical outcome after 12 months of treatment [187]. It is not clear however whether there is a direct effect of NTZ on microglia.

4.6.2 Anti-CD20 antibodies

There are multiple anti-CD20 monoclonal antibodies shown to ameliorate relapses in relapsing-remitting MS including rituximab, ocrelizumab, and ofatumumab [188]. However, ocrelizumab is the only anti-CD20 antibody that exerts beneficial effects in relapsing-remitting and also in primary progressive MS [189]. A subset of GM-CSF-producing memory B cells, more prevalent in MS patients than healthy controls, was shown to activate pro-inflammatory myeloid cells in vitro [190]. Following B-cell-depleting therapy in MS patients, the inflammatory myeloid response is diminished [190].

4.6.3 Alemtuzumab

Alemtuzumab is a monoclonal antibody that binds CD52 and effectively depletes CD52-expressing lymphocytes through antibody-dependent cell-mediated cytolysis. Both lymphocytes and myeloid cells express CD52; however, myeloid cells are more resistant to alemtuzumab-mediated cytolysis. Thus their numbers are not affected by treatment [191]. Neutrophils, however, express CD52 and are subject to lysis during alemtuzumab treatment [192], occasionally leading to severe neutropenia [193].

5. Conclusion

The contribution of myeloid cells to MS progression is now widely appreciated. Their persistent elevated presence in lesions and activated phenotype, regardless of tissue infiltration load, in both relapsing and progressive MS, suggest they play crucial roles in disease progression and chronicity. Although gaps in knowledge still exist, recent advances faciltated the efforts by researchers and clinicians to dissect the roles of each myeloid subset in the disease process.

Current therapeutics have broad activities or specifically target lymphocyte functions. In many instances, however, their efficacy stems from their direct or indirect effects on myeloid cell functions. Future research focusing on modulation of myeloid populations and their activities will prove useful for the design of novel therapeutics for MS patients.

Acknowledgements

National Multiple Sclerosis Society (RG-1701-26770) and Shriners Hospitals for Children (85114-NCA-18).

Conflict of interest

The authors declare no conflicts of interest.

Author details

Marilyn Wang[1,2], Sofia Caryotakis[1], Nagendra Kumar Rai[1,3], Alan Nguyen[1,3] and Athena M. Soulika[1,3*]

1 Shriners Hospital for Children—North America, Sacramento, USA

2 Department of Neurology, University of California, Davis School of Medicine, Sacramento, USA

3 Department of Dermatology, University of California, Davis School of Medicine, Sacramento, USA

*Address all correspondence to: asoulika@ucdavis.edu

References

[1] Goldmann T, Wieghofer P, Jordao MJ, Prutek F, Hagemeyer N, Frenzel K, et al. Origin, fate and dynamics of macrophages at central nervous system interfaces. Nature Immunology. 2016;**17**(7):797-805

[2] Mrdjen D, Pavlovic A, Hartmann FJ, Schreiner B, Utz SG, Leung BP, et al. High-dimensional single-cell mapping of central nervous system immune cells reveals distinct myeloid subsets in health, aging, and disease. Immunity. 2018;**48**(3):599

[3] Mundt S, Mrdjen D, Utz SG, Greter M, Schreiner B, Becher B. Conventional DCs sample and present myelin antigens in the healthy CNS and allow parenchymal T cell entry to initiate neuroinflammation. Science Immunology. 2019;**4**(31). pii: eaau8380

[4] Herz J, Filiano AJ, Smith A, Yogev N, Kipnis J. Myeloid cells in the central nervous system. Immunity. 2017;**46**(6):943-956

[5] Nayak D, Roth TL, McGavern DB. Microglia development and function. Annual Review of Immunology. 2014;**32**:367-402

[6] Schulz C, Gomez Perdiguero E, Chorro L, Szabo-Rogers H, Cagnard N, Kierdorf K, et al. A lineage of myeloid cells independent of Myb and hematopoietic stem cells. Science. 2012;**336**(6077):86-90

[7] Ginhoux F, Greter M, Leboeuf M, Nandi S, See P, Gokhan S, et al. Fate mapping analysis reveals that adult microglia derive from primitive macrophages. Science. 2010;**330**(6005):841-845

[8] Kierdorf K, Erny D, Goldmann T, Sander V, Schulz C, Perdiguero EG, et al. Microglia emerge from erythromyeloid precursors via Pu.1- and Irf8-dependent pathways. Nature Neuroscience. 2013;**16**(3):273-280

[9] Rymo SF, Gerhardt H, Wolfhagen Sand F, Lang R, Uv A, Betsholtz C. A two-way communication between microglial cells and angiogenic sprouts regulates angiogenesis in aortic ring cultures. PLoS One. 2011;**6**(1):e15846

[10] Hammond TR, Robinton D, Stevens B. Microglia and the brain: Complementary partners in development and disease. Annual Review of Cell and Developmental Biology. 2018;**34**:523-544

[11] Torres L, Danver J, Ji K, Miyauchi JT, Chen D, Anderson ME, et al. Dynamic microglial modulation of spatial learning and social behavior. Brain, Behavior, and Immunity. 2016;**55**:6-16

[12] Matcovitch-Natan O, Winter DR, Giladi A, Vargas Aguilar S, Spinrad A, Sarrazin S, et al. Microglia development follows a stepwise program to regulate brain homeostasis. Science. 2016;**353**(6301):aad8670

[13] Cunningham CL, Martinez-Cerdeno V, Noctor SC. Microglia regulate the number of neural precursor cells in the developing cerebral cortex. The Journal of Neuroscience. 2013;**33**(10):4216-4233

[14] Parkhurst CN, Yang G, Ninan I, Savas JN, Yates JR 3rd, Lafaille JJ, et al. Microglia promote learning-dependent synapse formation through brain-derived neurotrophic factor. Cell. 2013;**155**(7):1596-1609

[15] Paolicelli RC, Bolasco G, Pagani F, Maggi L, Scianni M, Panzanelli P, et al. Synaptic pruning by microglia is necessary for normal brain development. Science. 2011;**333**(6048):1456-1458

[16] Stevens B, Allen NJ, Vazquez LE, Howell GR, Christopherson KS, Nouri N, et al. The classical complement cascade mediates CNS synapse elimination. Cell. 2007;**131**(6):1164-1178

[17] Nandi S, Gokhan S, Dai XM, Wei S, Enikolopov G, Lin H, et al. The CSF-1 receptor ligands IL-34 and CSF-1 exhibit distinct developmental brain expression patterns and regulate neural progenitor cell maintenance and maturation. Developmental Biology. 2012;**367**(2):100-113

[18] Kierdorf K, Prinz M. Microglia in steady state. The Journal of Clinical Investigation. 2017;**127**(9):3201-3209

[19] Zhan Y, Paolicelli RC, Sforazzini F, Weinhard L, Bolasco G, Pagani F, et al. Deficient neuron-microglia signaling results in impaired functional brain connectivity and social behavior. Nature Neuroscience. 2014;**17**(3):400-406

[20] Marin-Teva JL, Dusart I, Colin C, Gervais A, van Rooijen N, Mallat M. Microglia promote the death of developing Purkinje cells. Neuron. 2004;**41**(4):535-547

[21] Araujo DM, Cotman CW. Basic FGF in astroglial, microglial, and neuronal cultures: Characterization of binding sites and modulation of release by lymphokines and trophic factors. The Journal of Neuroscience. 1992;**12**(5):1668-1678

[22] Nakajima K, Honda S, Tohyama Y, Imai Y, Kohsaka S, Kurihara T. Neurotrophin secretion from cultured microglia. Journal of Neuroscience Research. 2001;**65**(4):322-331

[23] Trang T, Beggs S, Salter MW. Brain-derived neurotrophic factor from microglia: A molecular substrate for neuropathic pain. Neuron Glia Biology. 2011;7(1):99-108

[24] De Biase LM, Schuebel KE, Fusfeld ZH, Jair K, Hawes IA, Cimbro R, et al. Local cues establish and maintain region-specific phenotypes of basal ganglia microglia. Neuron. 2017;**95**(2):341-356. e6

[25] Grabert K, Michoel T, Karavolos MH, Clohisey S, Baillie JK, Stevens MP, et al. Microglial brain region-dependent diversity and selective regional sensitivities to aging. Nature Neuroscience. 2016;**19**(3):504-516

[26] Butovsky O, Weiner HL. Microglial signatures and their role in health and disease. Nature Reviews. Neuroscience. 2018;**19**(10):622-635

[27] Hanisch UK. Functional diversity of microglia—How heterogeneous are they to begin with? Frontiers in Cellular Neuroscience. 2013;7:65

[28] Ransohoff RM, Cardona AE. The myeloid cells of the central nervous system parenchyma. Nature. 2010;**468**(7321):253-262

[29] Hammond TR, Dufort C, Dissing-Olesen L, Giera S, Young A, Wysoker A, et al. Single-cell RNA sequencing of microglia throughout the mouse lifespan and in the injured brain reveals complex cell-state changes. Immunity. 2019;**50**(1):253-271. e6

[30] Masuda T, Sankowski R, Staszewski O, Bottcher C, Amann L, Scheiwe C, et al. Spatial and temporal heterogeneity of mouse and human microglia at single-cell resolution. Nature. 2019;**566**(7744):388-392

[31] Huang Y, Xu Z, Xiong S, Sun F, Qin G, Hu G, et al. Repopulated microglia are solely derived from the proliferation of residual microglia after acute depletion. Nature Neuroscience. 2018;**21**(4):530-540

[32] Zhan L, Krabbe G, Du F, Jones I, Reichert MC, Telpoukhovskaia M,

et al. Proximal recolonization by self-renewing microglia re-establishes microglial homeostasis in the adult mouse brain. PLoS Biology. 2019;**17**(2):e3000134

[33] Cronk JC, Filiano AJ, Louveau A, Marin I, Marsh R, Ji E, et al. Peripherally derived macrophages can engraft the brain independent of irradiation and maintain an identity distinct from microglia. The Journal of Experimental Medicine. 2018;**215**(6):1627-1647

[34] Chitu V, Gokhan S, Nandi S, Mehler MF, Stanley ER. Emerging roles for CSF-1 receptor and its ligands in the nervous system. Trends in Neurosciences. 2016;**39**(6):378-393

[35] Wu S, Xue R, Hassan S, Nguyen TML, Wang T, Pan H, et al. Il34-Csf1r pathway regulates the migration and colonization of microglial precursors. Developmental Cell. 2018;**46**(5): 552-563 e4

[36] Buttgereit A, Lelios I, Yu X, Vrohlings M, Krakoski NR, Gautier EL, et al. Sall1 is a transcriptional regulator defining microglia identity and function. Nature Immunology. 2016;**17**(12):1397-1406

[37] Butovsky O, Jedrychowski MP, Moore CS, Cialic R, Lanser AJ, Gabriely G, et al. Identification of a unique TGF-beta-dependent molecular and functional signature in microglia. Nature Neuroscience. 2014;**17**(1):131-143

[38] Hickman SE, Kingery ND, Ohsumi TK, Borowsky ML, Wang LC, Means TK, et al. The microglial sensome revealed by direct RNA sequencing. Nature Neuroscience. 2013;**16**(12):1896-1905

[39] Jiang ZH, Peng J, Yang HL, Fu XL, Wang JZ, Liu L, et al. Upregulation and biological function of transmembrane protein 119 in osteosarcoma. Experimental & Molecular Medicine. 2017;**49**(5):e329

[40] Tanaka K, Inoue Y, Hendy GN, Canaff L, Katagiri T, Kitazawa R, et al. Interaction of Tmem119 and the bone morphogenetic protein pathway in the commitment of myoblastic into osteoblastic cells. Bone. 2012;**51**(1):158-167

[41] Tanaka K, Kaji H, Yamaguchi T, Kanazawa I, Canaff L, Hendy GN, et al. Involvement of the osteoinductive factors, Tmem119 and BMP-2, and the ER stress response PERK-eIF2alpha-ATF4 pathway in the commitment of myoblastic into osteoblastic cells. Calcified Tissue International. 2014;**94**(4):454-464

[42] Zheng P, Wang W, Ji M, Zhu Q, Feng Y, Zhou F, et al. TMEM119 promotes gastric cancer cell migration and invasion through STAT3 signaling pathway. OncoTargets and Therapy. 2018;**11**:5835-5844

[43] Bachstetter AD, Morganti JM, Jernberg J, Schlunk A, Mitchell SH, Brewster KW, et al. Fractalkine and CX 3 CR1 regulate hippocampal neurogenesis in adult and aged rats. Neurobiology of Aging. 2011;**32**(11):2030-2044

[44] Sellner S, Paricio-Montesinos R, Spiess A, Masuch A, Erny D, Harsan LA, et al. Microglial CX3CR1 promotes adult neurogenesis by inhibiting Sirt 1/p65 signaling independent of CX3CL1. Acta Neuropathologica Communications. 2016;**4**(1):102

[45] Vukovic J, Colditz MJ, Blackmore DG, Ruitenberg MJ, Bartlett PF. Microglia modulate hippocampal neural precursor activity in response to exercise and aging. The Journal of Neuroscience. 2012;**32**(19):6435-6443

[46] Fourgeaud L, Traves PG, Tufail Y, Leal-Bailey H, Lew ED, Burrola PG,

et al. TAM receptors regulate multiple features of microglial physiology. Nature. 2016;**532**(7598):240-244

[47] Hagemeyer N, Hanft KM, Akriditou MA, Unger N, Park ES, Stanley ER, et al. Microglia contribute to normal myelinogenesis and to oligodendrocyte progenitor maintenance during adulthood. Acta Neuropathologica. 2017;**134**(3):441-458

[48] Wlodarczyk A, Holtman IR, Krueger M, Yogev N, Bruttger J, Khorooshi R, et al. A novel microglial subset plays a key role in myelinogenesis in developing brain. The EMBO Journal. 2017;**36**(22):3292-3308

[49] Keaney J, Campbell M. The dynamic blood-brain barrier. The FEBS Journal. 2015;**282**(21):4067-4079

[50] Obermeier B, Daneman R, Ransohoff RM. Development, maintenance and disruption of the blood-brain barrier. Nature Medicine. 2013;**19**(12):1584-1596

[51] Lou N, Takano T, Pei Y, Xavier AL, Goldman SA, Nedergaard M. Purinergic receptor P2RY12-dependent microglial closure of the injured blood-brain barrier. Proceedings of the National Academy of Sciences of the United States of America. 2016;**113**(4):1074-1079

[52] Katsumoto A, Lu H, Miranda AS, Ransohoff RM. Ontogeny and functions of central nervous system macrophages. Journal of Immunology. 2014;**193**(6):2615-2621

[53] Checchin D, Sennlaub F, Levavasseur E, Leduc M, Chemtob S. Potential role of microglia in retinal blood vessel formation. Investigative Ophthalmology & Visual Science. 2006;**47**(8):3595-3602

[54] Liu C, Wu C, Yang Q, Gao J, Li L, Yang D, et al. Macrophages mediate the repair of brain vascular rupture through direct physical adhesion and mechanical traction. Immunity. 2016;**44**(5):1162-1176

[55] Kunis G, Baruch K, Miller O, Schwartz M. Immunization with a myelin-derived antigen activates the brain's choroid plexus for recruitment of immunoregulatory cells to the CNS and attenuates disease progression in a mouse model of ALS. The Journal of Neuroscience. 2015;**35**(16):6381-6393

[56] Prinz M, Erny D, Hagemeyer N. Ontogeny and homeostasis of CNS myeloid cells. Nature Immunology. 2017;**18**(4):385-392

[57] Reboldi A, Coisne C, Baumjohann D, Benvenuto F, Bottinelli D, Lira S, et al. C-C chemokine receptor 6-regulated entry of TH-17 cells into the CNS through the choroid plexus is required for the initiation of EAE. Nature Immunology. 2009;**10**(5):514-523

[58] Zeisel A, Munoz-Manchado AB, Codeluppi S, Lonnerberg P, La Manno G, Jureus A, et al. Brain structure. Cell types in the mouse cortex and hippocampus revealed by single-cell RNA-seq. Science. 2015;**347**(6226):1138-1142

[59] Waskow C, Liu K, Darrasse-Jeze G, Guermonprez P, Ginhoux F, Merad M, et al. The receptor tyrosine kinase Flt3 is required for dendritic cell development in peripheral lymphoid tissues. Nature Immunology. 2008;**9**(6):676-683

[60] Anandasabapathy N, Victora GD, Meredith M, Feder R, Dong B, Kluger C, et al. Flt3L controls the development of radiosensitive dendritic cells in the meninges and choroid plexus of the steady-state mouse brain. The Journal of Experimental Medicine. 2011;**208**(8):1695-1705

[61] Harpur CM, Kato Y, Dewi ST, Stankovic S, Johnson DN, Bedoui S, et al. Classical type 1 dendritic cells dominate priming of Th1 responses to herpes simplex virus type 1 skin infection. Journal of Immunology. 2019;**202**(3):653-663

[62] Lee CH, Chen JS, Chiu HC, Hong CH, Liu CY, Ta YC, et al. Differential activation behavior of dermal dendritic cells underlies the strain-specific Th1 responses to single epicutaneous immunization. Journal of Dermatological Science. 2016;**84**(3):248-257

[63] Collin M, Bigley V. Human dendritic cell subsets: An update. Immunology. 2018;**154**(1):3-20

[64] Langlet C, Tamoutounour S, Henri S, Luche H, Ardouin L, Gregoire C, et al. CD64 expression distinguishes monocyte-derived and conventional dendritic cells and reveals their distinct role during intramuscular immunization. Journal of Immunology. 2012;**188**(4):1751-1760

[65] Malissen B, Tamoutounour S, Henri S. The origins and functions of dendritic cells and macrophages in the skin. Nature Reviews. Immunology. 2014;**14**(6):417-428

[66] Theoharides TC. Mast cells: The immune gate to the brain. Life Sciences. 1990;**46**(9):607-617

[67] Silver R, Curley JP. Mast cells on the mind: New insights and opportunities. Trends in Neurosciences. 2013;**36**(9):513-521

[68] Kolaczkowska E, Kubes P. Neutrophil recruitment and function in health and inflammation. Nature Reviews. Immunology. 2013;**13**(3):159-175

[69] Geng S, Matsushima H, Okamoto T, Yao Y, Lu R, Page K, et al. Emergence, origin, and function of neutrophil-dendritic cell hybrids in experimentally induced inflammatory lesions in mice. Blood. 2013;**121**(10):1690-1700

[70] Christoffersson G, Vagesjo E, Vandooren J, Liden M, Massena S, Reinert RB, et al. VEGF-A recruits a proangiogenic MMP-9-delivering neutrophil subset that induces angiogenesis in transplanted hypoxic tissue. Blood. 2012;**120**(23):4653-4662

[71] Massena S, Christoffersson G, Vagesjo E, Seignez C, Gustafsson K, Binet F, et al. Identification and characterization of VEGF-A-responsive neutrophils expressing CD49d, VEGFR1, and CXCR4 in mice and humans. Blood. 2015;**126**(17):2016-2026

[72] Tourki B, Halade G. Leukocyte diversity in resolving and nonresolving mechanisms of cardiac remodeling. The FASEB Journal. 2017;**31**(10):4226-4239

[73] Cronk JC, Derecki NC, Ji E, Xu Y, Lampano AE, Smirnov I, et al. Methyl-CpG binding protein 2 regulates microglia and macrophage gene expression in response to inflammatory stimuli. Immunity. 2015;**42**(4):679-691

[74] Frossi B, Mion F, Sibilano R, Danelli L, Pucillo CEM. Is it time for a new classification of mast cells? What do we know about mast cell heterogeneity? Immunological Reviews. 2018;**282**(1):35-46

[75] Irani AM, Schwartz LB. Human mast cell heterogeneity. Allergy Proceedings. 1994;**15**(6):303-308

[76] Gupta K, Harvima IT. Mast cell-neural interactions contribute to pain and itch. Immunological Reviews. 2018;**282**(1):168-187

[77] Silverman AJ, Asarian L, Khalil M, Silver R. GnRH, brain mast cells and behavior. Progress in Brain Research. 2002;**141**:315-325

[78] Theoharides TC, Donelan J, Kandere-Grzybowska K, Konstantinidou A. The role of mast cells in migraine pathophysiology. Brain Research. Brain Research Reviews. 2005;**49**(1):65-76

[79] Crivellato E, Ribatti D. The mast cell: An evolutionary perspective. Biological Reviews of the Cambridge Philosophical Society. 2010;**85**(2):347-360

[80] Levy D. Migraine pain, meningeal inflammation, and mast cells. Current Pain and Headache Reports. 2009;**13**(3):237-240

[81] Chikahisa S, Kodama T, Soya A, Sagawa Y, Ishimaru Y, Sei H, et al. Histamine from brain resident MAST cells promotes wakefulness and modulates behavioral states. PLoS One. 2013;**8**(10):e78434

[82] Lenz KM, Pickett LA, Wright CL, Davis KT, Joshi A, McCarthy MM. Mast cells in the developing brain determine adult sexual behavior. The Journal of Neuroscience. 2018;**38**(37):8044-8059

[83] Wingerchuk DM, Lucchinetti CF, Noseworthy JH. Multiple sclerosis: Current pathophysiological concepts. Laboratory Investigation. 2001;**81**(3):263-281

[84] Lassmann H, Bradl M. Multiple sclerosis: Experimental models and reality. Acta Neuropathologica. 2017;**133**(2):223-244

[85] Constantinescu CS, Farooqi N, O'Brien K, Gran B. Experimental autoimmune encephalomyelitis (EAE) as a model for multiple sclerosis (MS). British Journal of Pharmacology. 2011;**164**(4):1079-1106

[86] Soulika AM, Lee E, McCauley E, Miers L, Bannerman P, Pleasure D. Initiation and progression of axonopathy in experimental autoimmune encephalomyelitis. The Journal of Neuroscience. 2009;**29**(47):14965-14979

[87] Chuluundorj D, Harding SA, Abernethy D, La Flamme AC. Expansion and preferential activation of the CD14(+)CD16(+) monocyte subset during multiple sclerosis. Immunology and Cell Biology. 2014;**92**(6):509-517

[88] Gjelstrup MC, Stilund M, Petersen T, Moller HJ, Petersen EL, Christensen T. Subsets of activated monocytes and markers of inflammation in incipient and progressed multiple sclerosis. Immunology and Cell Biology. 2018;**96**(2):160-174

[89] Karni A, Abraham M, Monsonego A, Cai G, Freeman GJ, Hafler D, et al. Innate immunity in multiple sclerosis: Myeloid dendritic cells in secondary progressive multiple sclerosis are activated and drive a proinflammatory immune response. Journal of Immunology. 2006;**177**(6):4196-4202

[90] Nuyts AH, Lee WP, Bashir-Dar R, Berneman ZN, Cools N. Dendritic cells in multiple sclerosis: Key players in the immunopathogenesis, key players for new cellular immunotherapies? Multiple Sclerosis. 2013;**19**(8):995-1002

[91] Dendrou CA, Fugger L, Friese MA. Immunopathology of multiple sclerosis. Nature Reviews. Immunology. 2015;**15**(9):545-558

[92] Popescu BF, Lucchinetti CF. Pathology of demyelinating diseases. Annual Review of Pathology. 2012;**7**:185-217

[93] Lucchinetti C, Bruck W, Parisi J, Scheithauer B, Rodriguez M, Lassmann H. Heterogeneity of multiple sclerosis lesions: Implications for the pathogenesis of demyelination. Annals of Neurology. 2000;**47**(6):707-717

[94] Mahad DH, Trapp BD, Lassmann H. Pathological mechanisms in progressive multiple sclerosis. Lancet Neurology. 2015;**14**(2):183-193

[95] Trapp BD, Peterson J, Ransohoff RM, Rudick R, Mork S, Bo L. Axonal transection in the lesions of multiple sclerosis. The New England Journal of Medicine. 1998;**338**(5):278-285

[96] Fischer MT, Sharma R, Lim JL, Haider L, Frischer JM, Drexhage J, et al. NADPH oxidase expression in active multiple sclerosis lesions in relation to oxidative tissue damage and mitochondrial injury. Brain. 2012;**135** (Pt 3):886-899

[97] Zrzavy T, Hametner S, Wimmer I, Butovsky O, Weiner HL, Lassmann H. Loss of 'homeostatic' microglia and patterns of their activation in active multiple sclerosis. Brain. 2017;**140**(7):1900-1913

[98] Boven LA, Van Meurs M, Van Zwam M, Wierenga-Wolf A, Hintzen RQ, Boot RG, et al. Myelin-laden macrophages are anti-inflammatory, consistent with foam cells in multiple sclerosis. Brain. 2006;**129**(Pt 2):517-526

[99] Fan X, Zhang H, Cheng Y, Jiang X, Zhu J, Jin T. Double roles of macrophages in human neuroimmune diseases and their animal models. Mediators of Inflammation. 2016;**2016**:8489251

[100] Gillen KM, Mubarak M, Nguyen TD, Pitt D. Significance and in vivo detection of iron-laden microglia in white matter multiple sclerosis lesions. Frontiers in Immunology. 2018;**9**:255

[101] Vogel DY, Vereyken EJ, Glim JE, Heijnen PD, Moeton M, van der Valk P, et al. Macrophages in inflammatory multiple sclerosis lesions have an intermediate activation status. Journal of Neuroinflammation. 2013;**10**:35

[102] Zhang Z, Zhang ZY, Schittenhelm J, Wu Y, Meyermann R, Schluesener HJ. Parenchymal accumulation of CD163+ macrophages/microglia in multiple sclerosis brains. Journal of Neuroimmunology. 2011;**237**(1-2):73-79

[103] Giles DA, Washnock-Schmid JM, Duncker PC, Dahlawi S, Ponath G, Pitt D, et al. Myeloid cell plasticity in the evolution of central nervous system autoimmunity. Annals of Neurology. 2018;**83**(1):131-141

[104] Mehta V, Pei W, Yang G, Li S, Swamy E, Boster A, et al. Iron is a sensitive biomarker for inflammation in multiple sclerosis lesions. PLoS One. 2013;**8**(3):e57573

[105] Popescu BF, Frischer JM, Webb SM, Tham M, Adiele RC, Robinson CA, et al. Pathogenic implications of distinct patterns of iron and zinc in chronic MS lesions. Acta Neuropathologica. 2017;**134**(1):45-64

[106] Hametner S, Wimmer I, Haider L, Pfeifenbring S, Bruck W, Lassmann H. Iron and neurodegeneration in the multiple sclerosis brain. Annals of Neurology. 2013;**74**(6):848-861

[107] Howell OW, Rundle JL, Garg A, Komada M, Brophy PJ, Reynolds R. Activated microglia mediate axoglial disruption that contributes to axonal injury in multiple sclerosis. Journal of Neuropathology and Experimental Neurology. 2010;**69**(10):1017-1033

[108] Melief J, Schuurman KG, van de Garde MD, Smolders J, van Eijk M, Hamann J, et al. Microglia in normal appearing white matter of multiple sclerosis are alerted but immunosuppressed. Glia. 2013;**61**(11):1848-1861

[109] Singh S, Metz I, Amor S, van der Valk P, Stadelmann C, Bruck W. Microglial nodules in early multiple sclerosis white matter

are associated with degenerating axons. Acta Neuropathologica. 2013;**125**(4):595-608

[110] Herranz E, Gianni C, Louapre C, Treaba CA, Govindarajan ST, Ouellette R, et al. Neuroinflammatory component of gray matter pathology in multiple sclerosis. Annals of Neurology. 2016;**80**(5):776-790

[111] Politis M, Giannetti P, Su P, Turkheimer F, Keihaninejad S, Wu K, et al. Increased PK11195 PET binding in the cortex of patients with MS correlates with disability. Neurology. 2012;**79**(6):523-530

[112] Abdelhak A, Weber MS, Tumani H. Primary progressive multiple sclerosis: Putting together the puzzle. Frontiers in Neurology. 2017;**8**:234

[113] Howell OW, Reeves CA, Nicholas R, Carassiti D, Radotra B, Gentleman SM, et al. Meningeal inflammation is widespread and linked to cortical pathology in multiple sclerosis. Brain. 2011;**134**(Pt 9):2755-2771

[114] Michailidou I, Naessens DM, Hametner S, Guldenaar W, Kooi EJ, Geurts JJ, et al. Complement C3 on microglial clusters in multiple sclerosis occur in chronic but not acute disease: Implication for disease pathogenesis. Glia. 2017;**65**(2):264-277

[115] Shemer A, Grozovski J, Tay TL, Tao J, Volaski A, Suss P, et al. Engrafted parenchymal brain macrophages differ from microglia in transcriptome, chromatin landscape and response to challenge. Nature Communications. 2018;**9**(1):5206

[116] Said A, Weindl G. Regulation of dendritic cell function in inflammation. Journal of Immunology Research. 2015;**2015**:743169

[117] Pierson ER, Wagner CA, Goverman JM. The contribution of neutrophils to CNS autoimmunity. Clinical Immunology. 2018;**189**:23-28

[118] Brinkmann V, Reichard U, Goosmann C, Fauler B, Uhlemann Y, Weiss DS, et al. Neutrophil extracellular traps kill bacteria. Science. 2004;**303**(5663):1532-1535

[119] Naegele M, Tillack K, Reinhardt S, Schippling S, Martin R, Sospedra M. Neutrophils in multiple sclerosis are characterized by a primed phenotype. Journal of Neuroimmunology. 2012;**242**(1-2):60-71

[120] Saadoun S, Waters P, MacDonald C, Bell BA, Vincent A, Verkman AS, et al. Neutrophil protease inhibition reduces neuromyelitis optica-immunoglobulin G-induced damage in mouse brain. Annals of Neurology. 2012;**71**(3):323-333

[121] Woodberry T, Bouffler SE, Wilson AS, Buckland RL, Brustle A. The emerging role of neutrophil granulocytes in multiple sclerosis. Journal of Clinical Medicine. 2018;**7**(12). pii: E511

[122] Kostic M, Dzopalic T, Zivanovic S, Zivkovic N, Cvetanovic A, Stojanovic I, et al. IL-17 and glutamate excitotoxicity in the pathogenesis of multiple sclerosis. Scandinavian Journal of Immunology. 2014;**79**(3):181-186

[123] Campbell SJ, Meier U, Mardiguian S, Jiang Y, Littleton ET, Bristow A, et al. Sickness behaviour is induced by a peripheral CXC-chemokine also expressed in multiple sclerosis and EAE. Brain, Behavior, and Immunity. 2010;**24**(5):738-746

[124] Ishizu T, Osoegawa M, Mei FJ, Kikuchi H, Tanaka M, Takakura Y, et al. Intrathecal activation of the IL-17/IL-8 axis in opticospinal multiple sclerosis. Brain. 2005;**128**(Pt 5):988-1002

[125] Rumble JM, Huber AK, Krishnamoorthy G, Srinivasan A,

Giles DA, Zhang X, et al. Neutrophil-related factors as biomarkers in EAE and MS. The Journal of Experimental Medicine. 2015;**212**(1):23-35

[126] Lock C, Hermans G, Pedotti R, Brendolan A, Schadt E, Garren H, et al. Gene-microarray analysis of multiple sclerosis lesions yields new targets validated in autoimmune encephalomyelitis. Nature Medicine. 2002;**8**(5):500-508

[127] Burt RK, Fassas A, Snowden J, van Laar JM, Kozak T, Wulffraat NM, et al. Collection of hematopoietic stem cells from patients with autoimmune diseases. Bone Marrow Transplantation. 2001;**28**(1):1-12

[128] Openshaw H, Lund BT, Kashyap A, Atkinson R, Sniecinski I, Weiner LP, et al. Peripheral blood stem cell transplantation in multiple sclerosis with busulfan and cyclophosphamide conditioning: Report of toxicity and immunological monitoring. Biology of Blood and Marrow Transplantation. 2000;**6**(5A):563-575

[129] Neumann J. Ueber das Vorkommen der sogenannten "Mastzellen" bei pathologischen Veränderungen des Gehirns. Archiv für pathologische Anatomie und Physiologie und für klinische Medicin. 1890;**122**(2):378-308

[130] Ibrahim MZ, Reder AT, Lawand R, Takash W, Sallouh-Khatib S. The mast cells of the multiple sclerosis brain. Journal of Neuroimmunology. 1996;**70**(2):131-138

[131] Olsson Y. Mast cells in plaques of multiple sclerosis. Acta Neurologica Scandinavica. 1974;**50**(5):611-618

[132] Toms R, Weiner HL, Johnson D. Identification of IgE-positive cells and mast cells in frozen sections of multiple sclerosis brains. Journal of Neuroimmunology. 1990;**30**(2-3):169-177

[133] Brown MA, Weinberg RB. Mast cells and innate lymphoid cells: Underappreciated players in CNS autoimmune demyelinating disease. Frontiers in Immunology. 2018;**9**:514

[134] Calabresi PA, Stone LA, Bash CN, Frank JA, McFarland HF. Interferon beta results in immediate reduction of contrast-enhanced MRI lesions in multiple sclerosis patients followed by weekly MRI. Neurology. 1997;**48**(5):1446-1448

[135] Jacobs LD, Cookfair DL, Rudick RA, Herndon RM, Richert JR, Salazar AM, et al. Intramuscular interferon beta-1a for disease progression in relapsing multiple sclerosis. The Multiple Sclerosis Collaborative Research Group (MSCRG). Annals of Neurology. 1996;**39**(3):285-294

[136] Guarda G, Braun M, Staehli F, Tardivel A, Mattmann C, Forster I, et al. Type I interferon inhibits interleukin-1 production and inflammasome activation. Immunity. 2011;**34**(2):213-223

[137] Ramgolam VS, Sha Y, Jin J, Zhang X, Markovic-Plese S. IFN-beta inhibits human Th17 cell differentiation. Journal of Immunology. 2009;**183**(8):5418-5427

[138] Prinz M, Schmidt H, Mildner A, Knobeloch KP, Hanisch UK, Raasch J, et al. Distinct and nonredundant in vivo functions of IFNAR on myeloid cells limit autoimmunity in the central nervous system. Immunity. 2008;**28**(5):675-686

[139] Bustamante MF, Nurtdinov RN, Rio J, Montalban X, Comabella M. Baseline gene expression signatures in monocytes from multiple sclerosis patients treated with interferon-beta. PLoS One. 2013;**8**(4):e60994

[140] Comabella M, Lunemann JD, Rio J, Sanchez A, Lopez C, Julia E, et al. A type I interferon signature in monocytes

is associated with poor response to interferon-beta in multiple sclerosis. Brain. 2009;**132**(Pt 12):3353-3365

[141] Zula JA, Green HC, Ransohoff RM, Rudick RA, Stark GR, van Boxel-Dezaire AH. The role of cell type-specific responses in IFN-beta therapy of multiple sclerosis. Proceedings of the National Academy of Sciences of the United States of America. 2011;**108**(49):19689-19694

[142] Hebb AL, Moore CS, Bhan V, Robertson GS. Effects of IFN-B on TRAIL and decoy receptor expression in different immune cell populations from MS patients with distinct disease subtypes. Autoimmune Disease. 2010;**2011**:485752

[143] Marckmann S, Wiesemann E, Hilse R, Trebst C, Stangel M, Windhagen A. Interferon-beta up-regulates the expression of co-stimulatory molecules CD80, CD86 and CD40 on monocytes: Significance for treatment of multiple sclerosis. Clinical and Experimental Immunology. 2004;**138**(3):499-506

[144] Wiesemann E, Deb M, Trebst C, Hemmer B, Stangel M, Windhagen A. Effects of interferon-beta on co-signaling molecules: Upregulation of CD40, CD86 and PD-L2 on monocytes in relation to clinical response to interferon-beta treatment in patients with multiple sclerosis. Multiple Sclerosis. 2008;**14**(2):166-176

[145] Sellebjerg F, Krakauer M, Limborg S, Hesse D, Lund H, Langkilde A, et al. Endogenous and recombinant type I interferons and disease activity in multiple sclerosis. PLoS One. 2012;7(6):e35927

[146] Gamrekelashvili J, Giagnorio R, Jussofie J, Soehnlein O, Duchene J, Briseno CG, et al. Regulation of monocyte cell fate by blood vessels mediated by Notch signalling. Nature Communications. 2016;7:12597

[147] Adriani M, Nytrova P, Mbogning C, Hassler S, Medek K, Jensen PEH, et al. Monocyte NOTCH2 expression predicts IFN-beta immunogenicity in multiple sclerosis patients. JCI Insight. 2018;**3**(11). pii: 99274

[148] Prod'homme T, Zamvil SS. The evolving mechanisms of action of glatiramer acetate. Cold Spring Harbor Perspectives in Medicine. 2019;**9**(2). pii: a029249

[149] Weber MS, Hohlfeld R, Zamvil SS. Mechanism of action of glatiramer acetate in treatment of multiple sclerosis. Neurotherapeutics. 2007;**4**(4):647-653

[150] Fridkis-Hareli M, Teitelbaum D, Gurevich E, Pecht I, Brautbar C, Kwon OJ, et al. Direct binding of myelin basic protein and synthetic copolymer 1 to class II major histocompatibility complex molecules on living antigen-presenting cells—Specificity and promiscuity. Proceedings of the National Academy of Sciences of the United States of America. 1994;**91**(11):4872-4876

[151] Teitelbaum D, Fridkis-Hareli M, Arnon R, Sela M. Copolymer 1 inhibits chronic relapsing experimental allergic encephalomyelitis induced by proteolipid protein (PLP) peptides in mice and interferes with PLP-specific T cell responses. Journal of Neuroimmunology. 1996;**64**(2):209-217

[152] Weber MS, Prod'homme T, Youssef S, Dunn SE, Rundle CD, Lee L, et al. Type II monocytes modulate T cell-mediated central nervous system autoimmune disease. Nature Medicine. 2007;**13**(8):935-943

[153] Kim HJ, Ifergan I, Antel JP, Seguin R, Duddy M, Lapierre Y, et al. Type 2 monocyte and microglia differentiation mediated by glatiramer acetate therapy in patients with multiple

sclerosis. Journal of Immunology. 2004;**172**(11):7144-7153

[154] Chuluundorj D, Harding SA, Abernethy D, La Flamme AC. Glatiramer acetate treatment normalized the monocyte activation profile in MS patients to that of healthy controls. Immunology and Cell Biology. 2017;**95**(3):297-305

[155] Hussien Y, Sanna A, Soderstrom M, Link H, Huang YM. Glatiramer acetate and IFN-beta act on dendritic cells in multiple sclerosis. Journal of Neuroimmunology. 2001;**121**(1-2):102-110

[156] Sellebjerg F, Hesse D, Limborg S, Lund H, Sondergaard HB, Krakauer M, et al. Dendritic cell, monocyte and T cell activation and response to glatiramer acetate in multiple sclerosis. Multiple Sclerosis. 2013;**19**(2):179-187

[157] van der Touw W, Kang K, Luan Y, Ma G, Mai S, Qin L, et al. Glatiramer acetate enhances myeloid-derived suppressor cell function via recognition of paired Ig-like receptor B. Journal of Immunology. 2018;**201**(6):1727-1734

[158] Mindur JE, Valenzuela RM, Yadav SK, Boppana S, Dhib-Jalbut S, Ito K. IL-27: A potential biomarker for responders to glatiramer acetate therapy. Journal of Neuroimmunology. 2017;**304**:21-28

[159] Lalive PH, Kreutzfeldt M, Devergne O, Metz I, Bruck W, Merkler D, et al. Increased interleukin-27 cytokine expression in the central nervous system of multiple sclerosis patients. Journal of Neuroinflammation. 2017;**14**(1):144

[160] Cohen JA, Barkhof F, Comi G, Hartung HP, Khatri BO, Montalban X, et al. Oral fingolimod or intramuscular interferon for relapsing multiple sclerosis. The New England Journal of Medicine. 2010;**362**(5):402-415

[161] Chun J, Kihara Y, Jonnalagadda D, Blaho VA. Fingolimod: Lessons learned and new opportunities for treating multiple sclerosis and other disorders. Annual Review of Pharmacology and Toxicology. 2019;**59**:149-170

[162] Brinkmann V, Billich A, Baumruker T, Heining P, Schmouder R, Francis G, et al. Fingolimod (FTY720): Discovery and development of an oral drug to treat multiple sclerosis. Nature Reviews. Drug Discovery. 2010;**9**(11):883-897

[163] Di Dario M, Colombo E, Govi C, De Feo D, Messina MJ, Romeo M, et al. Myeloid cells as target of fingolimod action in multiple sclerosis. Neurology: Neuroimmunology & Neuroinflammation. 2015;**2**(6):e157

[164] Durafourt BA, Lambert C, Johnson TA, Blain M, Bar-Or A, Antel JP. Differential responses of human microglia and blood-derived myeloid cells to FTY720. Journal of Neuroimmunology. 2011;**230**(1-2):10-16

[165] Hughes JE, Srinivasan S, Lynch KR, Proia RL, Ferdek P, Hedrick CC. Sphingosine-1-phosphate induces an antiinflammatory phenotype in macrophages. Circulation Research. 2008;**102**(8):950-958

[166] Thomas K, Sehr T, Proschmann U, Rodriguez-Leal FA, Haase R, Ziemssen T. Fingolimod additionally acts as immunomodulator focused on the innate immune system beyond its prominent effects on lymphocyte recirculation. Journal of Neuroinflammation. 2017;**14**(1):41

[167] Michell-Robinson MA, Moore CS, Healy LM, Osso LA, Zorko N, Grouza V, et al. Effects of fumarates on circulating and CNS myeloid cells in multiple sclerosis. Annals of Clinical Translational Neurology. 2016;**3**(1):27-41

[168] Foster CA, Howard LM, Schweitzer A, Persohn E, Hiestand PC, Balatoni B, et al. Brain penetration of the oral immunomodulatory drug FTY720 and its phosphorylation in the central nervous system during experimental autoimmune encephalomyelitis: Consequences for mode of action in multiple sclerosis. The Journal of Pharmacology and Experimental Therapeutics. 2007;**323**(2):469-475

[169] Linker RA, Lee DH, Ryan S, van Dam AM, Conrad R, Bista P, et al. Fumaric acid esters exert neuroprotective effects in neuroinflammation via activation of the Nrf2 antioxidant pathway. Brain. 2011;**134**(Pt 3):678-692

[170] Mills EA, Ogrodnik MA, Plave A, Mao-Draayer Y. Emerging understanding of the mechanism of action for dimethyl fumarate in the treatment of multiple sclerosis. Frontiers in Neurology. 2018;**9**:5

[171] Paraiso HC, Kuo PC, Curfman ET, Moon HJ, Sweazey RD, Yen JH, et al. Dimethyl fumarate attenuates reactive microglia and long-term memory deficits following systemic immune challenge. Journal of Neuroinflammation. 2018;**15**(1):100

[172] Schulze-Topphoff U, Varrin-Doyer M, Pekarek K, Spencer CM, Shetty A, Sagan SA, et al. Dimethyl fumarate treatment induces adaptive and innate immune modulation independent of Nrf2. Proceedings of the National Academy of Sciences of the United States of America. 2016;**113**(17):4777-4782

[173] Schilling S, Goelz S, Linker R, Luehder F, Gold R. Fumaric acid esters are effective in chronic experimental autoimmune encephalomyelitis and suppress macrophage infiltration. Clinical and Experimental Immunology. 2006;**145**(1):101-107

[174] Bar-Or A, Pachner A, Menguy-Vacheron F, Kaplan J, Wiendl H. Teriflunomide and its mechanism of action in multiple sclerosis. Drugs. 2014;**74**(6):659-674

[175] Bar-Or A. Teriflunomide (Aubagio(R)) for the treatment of multiple sclerosis. Experimental Neurology. 2014;**262** (Pt A):57-65

[176] Merrill JE, Hanak S, Pu SF, Liang J, Dang C, Iglesias-Bregna D, et al. Teriflunomide reduces behavioral, electrophysiological, and histopathological deficits in the Dark Agouti rat model of experimental autoimmune encephalomyelitis. Journal of Neurology. 2009;**256**(1):89-103

[177] Wostradowski T, Prajeeth CK, Gudi V, Kronenberg J, Witte S, Brieskorn M, et al. In vitro evaluation of physiologically relevant concentrations of teriflunomide on activation and proliferation of primary rodent microglia. Journal of Neuroinflammation. 2016;**13**(1):250

[178] Li L, Liu J, Delohery T, Zhang D, Arendt C, Jones C. The effects of teriflunomide on lymphocyte subpopulations in human peripheral blood mononuclear cells in vitro. Journal of Neuroimmunology. 2013;**265**(1-2):82-90

[179] Medina S, Sainz de la Maza S, Villarrubia N, Alvarez-Lafuente R, Costa-Frossard L, Arroyo R, et al. Teriflunomide induces a tolerogenic bias in blood immune cells of MS patients. Annals of Clinical Translational Neurology. 2019;**6**(2):355-363

[180] Polman CH, O'Connor PW, Havrdova E, Hutchinson M, Kappos L, Miller DH, et al. A randomized, placebo-controlled trial of natalizumab for relapsing multiple sclerosis. The New England Journal of Medicine. 2006;**354**(9):899-910

[181] Planas R, Jelcic I, Schippling S, Martin R, Sospedra M. Natalizumab treatment perturbs memory- and marginal zone-like B-cell homing in secondary lymphoid organs in multiple sclerosis. European Journal of Immunology. 2012;**42**(3):790-798

[182] Metz I, Radue EW, Oterino A, Kumpfel T, Wiendl H, Schippling S, et al. Pathology of immune reconstitution inflammatory syndrome in multiple sclerosis with natalizumab-associated progressive multifocal leukoencephalopathy. Acta Neuropathologica. 2012;**123**(2):235-245

[183] Kivisakk P, Francois K, Mbianda J, Gandhi R, Weiner HL, Khoury SJ. Effect of natalizumab treatment on circulating plasmacytoid dendritic cells: A cross-sectional observational study in patients with multiple sclerosis. PLoS One. 2014;**9**(7):e103716

[184] Painter MM, Atagi Y, Liu CC, Rademakers R, Xu H, Fryer JD, et al. TREM2 in CNS homeostasis and neurodegenerative disease. Molecular Neurodegeneration. 2015;**10**:43

[185] Kleinberger G, Yamanishi Y, Suarez-Calvet M, Czirr E, Lohmann E, Cuyvers E, et al. TREM2 mutations implicated in neurodegeneration impair cell surface transport and phagocytosis. Science Translational Medicine. 2014;**6**(243):243ra86

[186] Piccio L, Buonsanti C, Cella M, Tassi I, Schmidt RE, Fenoglio C, et al. Identification of soluble TREM-2 in the cerebrospinal fluid and its association with multiple sclerosis and CNS inflammation. Brain. 2008;**131** (Pt 11):3081-3091

[187] Ohrfelt A, Axelsson M, Malmestrom C, Novakova L, Heslegrave A, Blennow K, et al. Soluble TREM-2 in cerebrospinal fluid from patients with multiple sclerosis treated with natalizumab or mitoxantrone. Multiple Sclerosis. 2016;**22**(12):1587-1595

[188] Greenfield AL, Hauser SL. B-cell therapy for multiple sclerosis: Entering an era. Annals of Neurology. 2018;**83**(1):13-26

[189] Montalban X, Hauser SL, Kappos L, Arnold DL, Bar-Or A, Comi G, et al. Ocrelizumab versus placebo in primary progressive multiple sclerosis. The New England Journal of Medicine. 2017;**376**(3):209-220

[190] Li R, Rezk A, Miyazaki Y, Hilgenberg E, Touil H, Shen P, et al. Proinflammatory GM-CSF-producing B cells in multiple sclerosis and B cell depletion therapy. Science Translational Medicine. 2015;**7**(310):310ra166

[191] Rao SP, Sancho J, Campos-Rivera J, Boutin PM, Severy PB, Weeden T, et al. Human peripheral blood mononuclear cells exhibit heterogeneous CD52 expression levels and show differential sensitivity to alemtuzumab mediated cytolysis. PLoS One. 2012;**7**(6):e39416

[192] Ambrose LR, Morel AS, Warrens AN. Neutrophils express CD52 and exhibit complement-mediated lysis in the presence of alemtuzumab. Blood. 2009;**114**(14):3052-3055

[193] Baker D, Giovannoni G, Schmierer K. Marked neutropenia: Significant but rare in people with multiple sclerosis after alemtuzumab treatment. Multiple Sclerosis and Related Disorders. 2017;**18**:181-183

Section 3

Diagnosis

Chapter 3

Diagnosis of Multiple Sclerosis

Joyce Pauline Joseph

Abstract

Multiple sclerosis (MS) is a chronic inflammatory demyelinating disorder of the central nervous system. Although there are no pathognomonic features to confirm the diagnosis of this immune-mediated disease, a constellation of clinical, radiological, and immune studies can ensure the clinician gets a more definitive diagnosis. Criteria have been made every few years based on research to clinch the diagnosis. The most recent criteria which are the McDonald criteria have been formed in 2001 and revised in 2005, 2010, and 2017. Most criteria are to be used only as a guide to facilitate the diagnosis of multiple sclerosis. Advances in demyelinating disorders will require diagnostic criteria to be revised every few years with scientists hoping for a more definitive and confirmative diagnosis. The cardinal features for diagnosis are dissemination in time and space. There should be no other possible explanation to the clinical features.

Keywords: multiple sclerosis, diagnosis, criteria, dissemination in time, dissemination in space

1. Introduction

Multiple sclerosis is an immune-mediated disease involving the central nervous system predominantly affecting the brain, spinal cord, and optic nerves. There is no gold standard or pathognomonic features that can distinguish MS from other neurological conditions with multiple anatomical site involvement. A comprehensive history obtained from the patient, clinical examination with the support of laboratory investigations with is required to assist in the diagnosis of MS. The key to diagnosis has always been dissemination in time, which translates into different time interval of clinical relapse, and dissemination of space, which is a variable anatomical site in the central nervous system. Hence difference in time and neuroanatomical site is essential. Several criteria have been created over the last several decades such as Schumacher criteria, [1], Poser criteria [2], and McDonald criteria [3–5]. McDonald criteria has been first established in 2001 and revised in 2005, 2010, and 2017. Revisions are necessary due to evolving research and advances in the field of demyelinating diseases. Researchers in neuroimmunology diseases concurred the diagnosis of MS could be made earlier and can be used for paediatric population and Asian patients [5]. Investigations are done for diagnosis of MS to ensure there are no other possible explanations for the clinical and radiological presentation. As the patient can be subjected to lifelong immune modulators and immunosuppressant, it is highly essential to ensure diagnosis is made accurately and possible differentials are monitored during follow-up. A clinician's job does not end with establishing diagnosis and instituting treatment. Careful surveillance is necessary to ensure we are in the right track as regards to the diagnosis. Misdiagnosis could still occur, and therefore it must be addressed, and measures should be undertaken to minimise them.

2. Making the diagnosis: symptoms and signs

Awareness about MS is crucial for the patient to seek attention, and to ask for a second opinion when necessary is important both for patients and healthcare providers. A good history with a knowledge of common presentations and bearing in mind neuroanatomical sites involved will be valuable in coming to a conclusion, and focused investigations will be needed. Knowledge of subtypes and classification will be helpful to the clinician.

Four subtypes of multiple sclerosis are used [6].

Active or disease activity is measured by clinical relapses and MRI evidence of contrast-enhanced lesion or new or enlarging lesion on T2-weighted images by annual clinical assessment.

Progression-progressive disability by annual clinical assessment

If no annual assessment is done, it is called indeterminate.

- Clinically isolated syndrome
    - Active
    - Not active
- Relapsing-remitting multiple sclerosis
    - Active
    - Not active
- Primary progressive disease
    - Active with progression
    - Active but without progression
    - Not active but with progression
    - Not active and without progression
- Secondary progressive disease
    - Active with progression
    - Active but without progression

2.1 Optic nerve

Optic nerve involvements are common and often the first presentation in multiple sclerosis [7]. The severity can vary from being asymptomatic to severe visual loss, and recovery could be complete, partial, or no resolution. The symptoms could begin as pain behind the eye and evolve into visual impairment in the centre of the eye and may worsen till visual acuity is lost. Diminished colour appreciation or dyschromatopsia may be seen. The pain associated with ON tends to progress over days. Visual improvement may occur in 3–8 weeks, and most visual recovery occurs within the first 6 months but can continue for up to 1 year after the acute event [8–12]. However, many patients may experience residual and variable visual complaints and dysfunction after recovery. Examination on optic neuritis could reveal no abnormalities, and deficits are present; there may be disc selling, fine haemorrhages, impaired visual acuity, central or centrocecal oedema, relative afferent pupillary defect or Marcus Gunn pupil, impaired colour vision, and pale optic discs [11]. Phosphenes, which are an experience of bright flashes of light without light entering the eye, Uhthoff's phenomenon where there is brief blurring of vision during physical exercise [13].

2.2 Spinal cord

Numbness and weakness of upper and or lower limbs are presentations seen in spinal cord lesions in MS [14]. Cord lesions also come with urinary incontinence, frequency, and urinary retention depending on the level and severity involved. Constipation and diarrhoea could relate to bowel dysfunction. The symptoms are of corticospinal tract lesion; a clear sensory level might guide the clinician to focus on a cord lesion rather than a peripheral lesion due to a lower motor neuron lesion. Clinical assessment may reveal increased tone, monoparesis, hemiparesis and quadriparesis, abnormal cutaneous and sensory deficit, and sphincter disturbance [14]. The clinical diagnosis involving the cord is called myelitis.

2.3 Brainstem

Double vision, speech difficulty, swallowing difficulty, nausea, vomiting, hiccups, vertigo, unsteadiness, and weakness of limbs are symptoms seen in brainstem lesions. Examination would reveal nystagmus, ophthalmoplegia, dysarthria, and facial weakness [14]. Cranial nerve deficits involving III–XII may be seen. Cerebellar connection with the brainstem can cause dysdiadochokinesia, dysmetria, and ataxia [15]. Brainstem lesions could also cause respiratory failure and locked-in syndrome. Localization of the neuroanatomical site can be judged based on the symptoms prior to neuroimaging.

2.4 Cerebellum

Unsteadiness involving upper and lower limbs, gait instability, and dysarthria are common symptoms seen in structures involving the cerebellum. Tremors, which are either due to cerebellar or thalamic involvement, could occur, and they result in tremor affecting limbs, trunk, and vocal cord, and head. Types of tremors are intention, postural, rest, and rubral (Alistair [16]). Cerebellar signs will be evident with a significant involvement of the cerebellum. A pure cerebellar syndrome is rare and other causes must be investigated. Tremors in cerebellar involvement affect arms, legs, head, and trunk in descending order of frequency. Face, tongue, and jaw were not affected in a study done by Alusi et al. [17].

2.5 Cerebrum

Symptoms involving the cerebral hemispheres correlate the site of lesion such as the parietal, temporal, frontal, and occipital lobes. Symptoms are right- or left-sided hemianaesthesia, hemiparesis, hemiplegia, or monoplegia and visual symptoms due to visual field defect. Aphasia or dysphasia and epilepsy are rare symptoms noted in MS [13].

2.6 Symptoms of multiple sclerosis in chronic disease

Spasticity, cognitive dysfunction, fatigue, affective disorders, and sexual dysfunction are normally seen in chronic disease [13]. An in-depth history during the first clinical assessment is a valuable asset to establishing the diagnosis.

3. Investigations in MS

3.1 Blood investigations

There are no blood investigations that are pathognomonic for the diagnosis of multiple sclerosis. However, in order to rule out other neurological conditions that can mimic MS, a complete workout is necessary. Screening for connective tissue diseases such as Systemic Lupus Erythematosus, antiphospholipid antibody, retroviral screen, other autoimmune condition such as thyroid disease, infectious diseases, Lyme disease and angiotensin converting enzyme are necessary [18].

3.2 Lumbar puncture

Lumbar puncture for CSF analysis is required as it can further assist in the diagnosis as its presence reveals a risk of developing MS in patients with clinically isolated syndrome [3, 5, 19]. In 2017, cerebrospinal fluid (CSF) is done to look for oligoclonal band and immunoglobulin G (IgG), and a parallel serum sample need to be taken as no OCB production is noted in the blood in multiple sclerosis. Oligoclonal band and immunoglobulin G are indicative of intrathecal inflammation which is B cell modulated from plasma cells seen in CNS inflammatory disease [20]. Distinctive CSF analysis will disclose slightly raised leucocyte count, B cells, or plasma cells in cytological analysis and raised IgG synthesis [21]. Oligoclonal band will be highly helpful in the event of other clinical features that are not diagnostic, and furthermore it depicts dissemination in space. Lumbar puncture is recommended in the following situations [5]:

- When clinical and MRI evidence is inadequate to make diagnosis of multiple sclerosis, especially if treatment is considered

- When there are atypical features of clinically isolated syndrome and in population where MS is less common such as children, older individuals, or non-white populations

The Panel on Diagnosis of Multiple Sclerosis [5] cautions diagnosis of multiple sclerosis early on in the disease and in children when OCB is negative in atypical clinical, radiological, or OCB findings.

There are two methods of analysing the CSF for oligoclonal band agarose gel electrophoresis/Coomasie Blue Staining and isoelectric focus/silver staining [22]. Oligoclonal bands are positive in up to 95% of patients with clinically definite multiple sclerosis.

3.3 Evoked potentials

Evoked potentials are electrophysiological tests done to look for evidence of silent lesions [23]. Abnormal or slowing of electrical conduction along the central nervous system pathway can be detected even when there are no obvious clinical features seen. Visual evoked potentials are visual stimulation, which consists high contrast black and white checkerboard where these squares, are changed places and response to this reversal is recorded. Delayed waveform depicts an optic nerve lesion. Brainstem evoked potentials are when auditory stimulations in the form of clicks are given for a response obtained from the brainstem. It assesses lower brainstem auditory pathway. The BAEP are abnormal when demyelination involves brainstem. Somatosensory evoked potentials are obtained when stimulation from the peripheral nerves in the upper limbs produces a response. An abnormal response could translate to demyelination within the central fibres of dorsal column-medial lemniscal pathways. Evoked potentials may not be useful with advances in MRI techniques and oligoclonal band, and they have not been included in McDonald criteria 2017.

3.4 Magnetic resonance imaging

Magnetic resonance imaging (MRI) is a neuroimaging of choice for diagnosis of MS and plays a key role in research, surveillance, and treatment. Although the McDonald criteria denote that two clinical attacks depicting dissemination in time and space are sufficient to make a diagnosis, neurologists and neurologist with interest in MS would require a baseline MRI to confirm diagnosis and for surveillance. White matter lesions in the MRI are characteristic with typical juxtacortical, cortical; periventricular, brainstem and spinal cord lesions are required. MRI protocols used in MS are spin echo T2 weighted, fluid-attenuated inversion recovery. The Consortium of MS Centres revised and updated guidelines for MRI ([24], www.mscare.org/mri).

3.4.1 MRI protocols adapted from the Consortium of MS Centers

Baseline studies for patients with a clinically isolated syndrome (CIS) and/or suspected MS:

- Brain MRI protocol with gadolinium at baseline and to establish dissemination in time

- Spinal cord MRI if myelitis, insufficient features on brain MRI to support diagnosis, or age > 40 years with nonspecific brain MRI findings

- A cervical cord MRI performed simultaneously with the brain MRI could have prognostic value in the evaluation of CIS patients with or without myelitis and would reduce the number of patients requiring a subsequent MRI appointment

- Orbital MRI if severe optic neuritis with poor recovery

Timing of a follow-up brain MRI protocol for patients with a CIS and/or suspected MS to look for evidence of dissemination in time (i.e. new T2 lesions or gadolinium-enhancing lesions):

- 6–12 months for high-risk CIS (e.g. $\geq$ 2 ovoid lesions on first MRI)

- 12–24 months for low-risk CIS (i.e. normal brain MRI) and/or uncertain clinical syndrome with suspicious brain MRI features (e.g. radiologic isolated syndrome [RIS])

Timing of brain MRI protocol for patients with an established diagnosis of MS:

- No recent prior imaging available (e.g. patient with established diagnosis of MS and new to your clinical practice)
- Postpartum to establish a new baseline
- Prior to starting or switching disease-modifying therapy
- Approximately 6–12 months after switching disease-modifying therapy to establish a new baseline on the new therapy
- Every 1–2 years while on disease-modifying therapy to assess for subclinical disease activity (i.e. new T2 lesions or gadolinium-enhancing lesions). Less frequent MRI scans required in clinically stable patients after 2–3 years of stable treatment (gadolinium-based contrast optional)
- Unexpected clinical deterioration or reassessment of original diagnosis (gadolinium-based contrast recommended)
- The use of gadolinium-based contrast agents is helpful but not essential for detecting subclinical disease activity because new T2 MS lesions can be identified on well-performed standardized MR imaging unless there is a large T2 lesion burden, which may obscure new T2 lesion activity.

4. Diagnosis of MS with McDonald criteria

The International Panel on Diagnosis of Multiple Sclerosis consists of 30 members of European, American, and Asian representatives who are experts in their field, met in 2016 and 2017 to revise and formulate a new guideline based on advances on MS. The criteria are to be used only in the setting of clinically isolated syndrome to diagnose MS and progressive MS [5].

4.1 Optical coherence tomography

Optical coherence tomography (OCT) is a noninvasive cross-sectional imaging in biological systems [26]. OCT assesses the peripapillary area of the retina. Retinal nerve fibre layer and ganglion cell layer thickness loss affects visual function, disability, and magnetic resonance imaging. OCT angiography is a new technique under study in MS [27]. Retinal nerve fibre thinning is seen in multiple sclerosis, and OCT is able to measure the loss. Fundoscopy is the clinical parallel of OCT.

5. Common differential diagnosis

Clinicians should bear in mind multiple sclerosis mimickers to ensure there is no other possible explanation. Common differentials are connective tissue disease such as systemic lupus erythematosus and antiphospholipid antibody syndrome. Neuromyelitis optical spectrum disorder, which was previously known as Devic's disease, is an immune-mediated disorder that can be distinguished, from MS by typical MRI lesions and/or anti-aquaporin 4 antibody. Other conditions are acute disseminated meningoencephalitis, small vessel disease, and Susac's syndrome.

5.1 Neuromyelitis optica spectrum disorder

Neuromyelitis optica spectrum disorder is often considered as a differential of MS. It was considered as a part and spectrum of Multiple sclerosis, till Aquaporin 4 antibody serum antibodies [28, 29] that target the water channel aquaporin 4 was considered in the pathogenesis of NMOSD. It is essential to differentiate multiple sclerosis and NMOSD as the treatment differs in both, and some treatment could be harmful.

Diagnostic criteria for NMOSD[30].

Diagnostic criteria for NMOSD with AQP4-IgG

1. At least one core clinical characteristic

2. Positive test for AQP4-IgG using best available detection method (cell-based assay strongly recommended)

3. Exclusion of alternative diagnoses

Diagnostic criteria for NMOSD without AQP4-IgG or unknown AQP4-IgG status:

1. At least two core clinical characteristic occurring as a result of one or more clinical attacks and meeting all of the following requirement:

2. At least one core clinical characteristic must be optic neuritis, acute myelitis with LETM, or area postrema syndrome

3. Dissemination in space (two or more core clinical characteristics)

4. Fulfilment of additional MRI requirements, as applicable

5. Negative test for AQP4-IgG using the best available detection method or testing unavailable

6. Exclusion of alternative diagnoses

Core clinical characteristics:

1. Optic neuritis

2. Acute myelitis

3. Area postrema syndrome: episode of otherwise unexplained hiccups or nausea and vomiting

4. Acute brainstem syndrome

5. Symptomatic narcolepsy or acute diencephalic clinical syndrome with NMOSD-typical diencephalic MRI lesions

Symptomatic cerebral syndrome with NMOSD-typical brain lesions

Additional MRI requirements for NMOSD without AQP4-IgG or unknown AQP4-IgG status:

- Acute optic neuritis
    - Requires brain MRI showing
    - Normal findings or only nonspecific white matter lesions, OR
    - Optic nerve MRI with T2-hyperintense lesion, or T1-weighted gadolinium-enhancing lesion extending over 1/2 optic nerve length or involving optic chiasm
- Acute myelitis: requires associated intramedullary MRI lesion extending over three or more contiguous segments (LETM) OR three or more contiguous segments of focal spinal cord atrophy in patients with history compatible with acute myelitis
- Area postrema syndrome: requires associated dorsal medulla/area postrema lesions
- Acute brainstem syndrome: requires associated periependymal brainstem lesions.

5.2 MOG antibody disease

Seronegative NMOSD patients have been associated with MOG antibody disease, which is a myelin oligodendrocyte glycoprotein and which is found only in the central nervous system. Myelin oligodendrocyte glycoprotein is a small part of myelin [31]. MOG can be found in extracellular surface of myelin sheaths and oligodendrocytes. MOG antibodies were seen in several demyelinating diseases of the central nervous system disorders [32, 33]. MOG antibody disease tends to favour women, which is one third of patients (**Figure 1**).

B-cell activation is the strongest element seen in central nervous system of multiple sclerosis patients. Central nervous system-directed antibodies are produced in the periphery in neuromyelitis optica and myelin oligodendrocyte glycoprotein antibody disease. MRZ reaction is antibodies against measles, rubella, and varicella zoster (**Tables 1–3**).

5.3 Acute disseminated encephalomyelitis

Acute disseminated encephalomyelitis (ADEM) is a central nervous system-demyelinating disease predominantly involving children and young adults. It has been noted in adults and elderly; it follows vaccination and postinfectious state. It is commonly monophasic and rarely multiphasic in nature, and it can involve the brain, spinal cord, and optic nerves as in multiple sclerosis. Fever, malaise, myalgias, headache, nausea, and vomiting can precede neurological symptoms of ADEM, which can begin 4–21 days after the antecedent event. Clinical features of ADEM are the development of a focal or multifocal neurological disorder which could be encephalopathy, coma, and focal and multifocal neurological signs like hemiparesis, cranial nerve palsies, paraparesis, meningismus, ataxia, movement disorders, and seizure [36]. The International Paediatric Multiple Sclerosis Study Group (IPMSSG) [37] proposed consensus definitions for paediatric-acquired

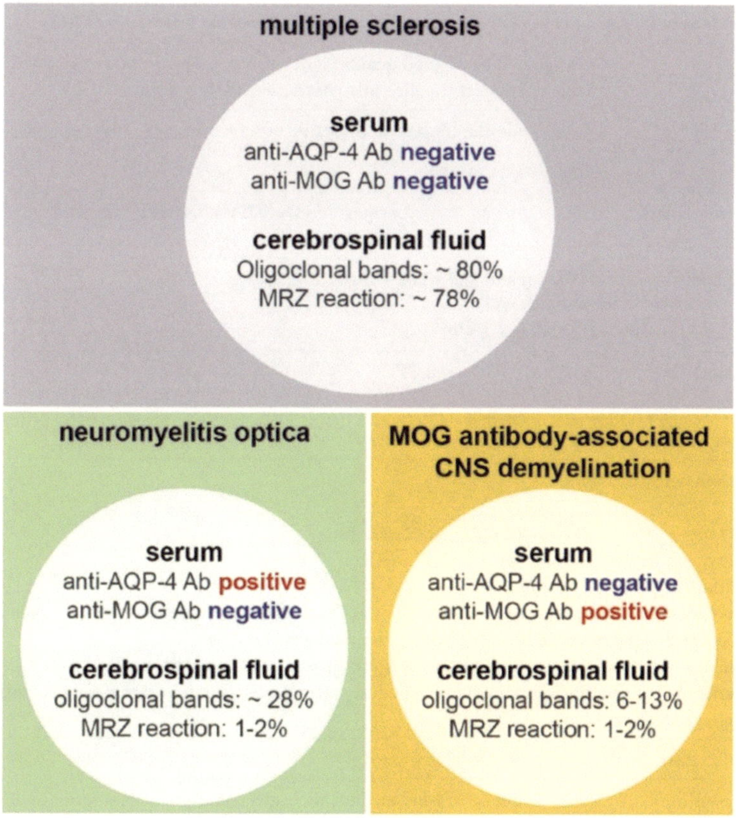

Figure 1.
Biomarkers in Multiple sclerosis, Neuromyelitis Optica Spectrum Disorder and MOG antibody disease. MRZ reaction are antibodies against measles, rubella and varicella zoster. (Adapted from [34]).

demyelinating disorders of the CNS to clarify the terminology for demyelination disease, and this was further updated in 2013 [38]. ADEM criteria require the following:

Monophasic ADEM:

i. A first polyfocal clinical neurological event with presumed inflammatory cause

ii. Encephalopathy that cannot be explained by fever is present

iii. No new clinical or radiological evidence of a new event suggestive of ADEM after 3 months

Multiphasic ADEM

i. A new onset of ADEM in 3 or more months after the primary event

ii. A new onset or reappearance of ADEM linked to previous clinical or radiological event involving the central nervous system

iii. Time of symptom onset in relation to steroids has no relevance

ADEM should be a diagnosis of exclusion and should be differentiated from multiple sclerosis from its clinical and radiological profile.

Protocol 1: Standardised brain MRI protocol (diagnosis and routine follow-up of MS)	
Field strength	Scans should be of good quality, with adequate signal-noise ratio (SNR) and spatial resolution (in-slice pixel resolution of ≤1 × 1 mm)
Scan prescription	Use the subcallosal plane to prescribe or reformat axial oblique slices
Coverage	Whole brain coverage
Slice thickness and gap	≤ 3 mm, no gap (for 2D acquisition Or 3D1 reconstruction)
Core sequences	2D/3D sagittal and Axial FLAIR1,2. 2D/3D axial T21 Axial 2D DWI3 3D IR-Prep GE4 T1
Gadolinium5 (as required)	Post-gad 2D/3D axial T1
Additional sequences	Susceptibility-weighted imaging (SWI). Pre-gad 2D/3D axial T1
Axial proton density	

1. 3D acquisition should be isotropic ≤1 × 1 × 1 mm
2. Fluid attenuated inversion recovery (FLAIR)
3. Diffusion-weighted imaging (DWI)
4. Inversion recovery-prepared gradient echo (IR-Prep GE); magnetization-prepared rapid acquisition gradient echo or MP-RAGE; turbo field echo Or TFE
5. Single dose of gadolinium-based contrast agent as required (note that the FLAIR Or T2 may be performed during the 5-minute minimum delay after gadolinium injection before acquiring the post-gadolinium T1)

Protocol 2: PML surveillance brain MRI protocol	
Field strength	Scans should be of good quality, with adequate signal-noise ratio (SNR) and resolution (in-slice pixel resolution of ≤1 × 1 mm)
Scan prescription	Use the subcallosal plane to prescribe or reformat axial oblique slices
Coverage	Whole brain coverage
Core sequences1	2D/3D sagittal and axial FLAIR2 axial 2D DWI3
Gadolinium (can be helpful) 4	Post-gad 2D/3D axial T1
Additional sequences	DWI
	2D/3D axial T2
	3D IR-Prep GE5 T1
	Pre-gad 2D/3D axial T1. Axial proton density
Slice thickness and gap	< 3 mm, no gap (for 2D acquisition or 3D reconstruction)

1. Typical PML lesions may appear hyperintense on FLAIR, hypointense on T1, and high signal intensity on DWI
2. Fluid attenuated inversion recovery (FLAIR)
3. Diffusion-weighted imaging (DWI)
4. Less than 50% of PML lesions will show contrast enhancement
5. Inversion recovery-prepared gradient echo (IR-Prep GE); magnetization-prepared rapid acquisition gradient echo or MP-RAGE; turbo field echo or TFE

Protocol 3: Spinal cord MRI protocol	
Field strength	Scans should be of good quality, with adequate signal-noise ratio (SNR) and resolution (in-slice pixel resolution of ≤1 × 1 mm)
Coverage	Cervical cord coverage1
Core sequences	Two of the following: sagittal T2

	Proton density STIR2
	T1-PSIR3
	Axial T2/T2* through lesions
Slice thickness and gap	Sagittal: <3 mm, no gap. Axial: <5 Mm, no gap
Additional sequences	Sagittal T1
	Post-gad T14 (sag, axial)
	Axial T2/T2* entire cervical cord 3D IR-Prep GE5 T1

1. Thoracic and conus coverage recommended if symptoms localize to this region to rule out an alternate diagnosis
2. Short tau inversion recovery (STIR)
3. Phase-sensitive T1 inversion recovery (PSIR)
4. No additional gadolinium necessary if cord examination immediately follows gadolinium-enhanced brain MRI
5. IR-Prep GE (inversion recovery-prepared gradient echo); magnetization-prepared rapid acquisition gradient echo or MP-RAGE; turbo field echo or TFE

Protocol 4: Orbit MRI protocol

- May be clinically indicated to confirm optic neuritis and rule out compressive lesions
- Recommended sequences include coronal STIR or fat-suppressed T2 and a post-gadolinium fat-suppressed T1 with a section thickness of ≤2 Mm, with coverage to include the optic chiasm
- Optional sequences may include axial/coronal pre-gadolinium fat-sat T1, axial fat-sat T2 or STIR, and axial post-gad fat-sat T1

Recommendations for communication
MRI requisition:
The clinician should provide on the request for the standardized MRI brain and/or spinal cord protocol:

- Clinical questions to be addressed *diagnosis

*Monitoring for management decision

- Relevant clinical history and physical examination findings
- Current MS disease-modifying treatment and JC virus status if on natalizumab
- If known, date and place of previous examinations

MRI report:
Standardised nomenclature/terminology should be used and include:

1. Description of findings

    - *Lesion type, location, size, shape, character, number for diagnostic

Scan

    - *CIS diagnostic scan: whether meets current MRI dissemination in space or dissemination in time criteria
    - *Qualitative assessment of T2 and brain volume/atrophy

2. MS monitoring or CIS follow-up: comparison with previous studies (new lesions, atrophy)
3. Interpretation (typical for MS, atypical for MS, not MS) and differential diagnosis, if appropriate

Note: structured reports can be helpful (Alessandrino et al., Ajr, 2018; Dickerson et al., J Am Coll Radiol 2017).
Recommendations:
*Studies should be stored in a DICOM format.
*Copies of MRI studies should be retained permanently and be available.
*It is strongly recommended for patients to keep their own studies on
Portable digital media

Table 1.
MRI protocols (Adapted from [25]).

National Multiple Sclerosis Society

2017 McDonald Criteria for the Diagnosis of Multiple Sclerosis

ECTRIMS — European Committee for Treatment and Research in Multiple Sclerosis

Diagnosis of MS requires elimination of more likely diagnoses and demonstration of dissemination of lesions in the CNS in space and time. See Lancet Neurology paper* for details.

CLINICAL PRESENTATION	ADDITIONAL DATA NEEDED TO MAKE MS DIAGNOSIS
...in a person with a typical attack/CIS at onset	(see KEY below for definitions)
• ≥2 attacks and objective clinical evidence of ≥2 lesions • ≥2 attacks and objective clinical evidence of 1 lesion with historical evidence of prior attack involving lesion in different location	None. Dissemination in space (**DIS**) and dissemination in time (**DIT**) have been met.
• ≥2 attacks and objective clinical evidence of 1 lesion	**One** of these criteria: – **DIS**: additional clinical attack implicating different CNS site – **DIS**: ≥1 symptomatic or asymptomatic MS-typical T2 lesions in ≥2 areas of CNS: periventricular, juxtacortical/cortical, infratentorial or spinal cord
• 1 attack and objective clinical evidence of ≥2 lesions	**One** of these criteria: – **DIT**: additional clinical attack – **DIT**: simultaneous presence of both enhancing and non-enhancing symptomatic or asymptomatic MS-typical MRI lesions – **DIT**: new T2 or enhancing MRI lesion compared to baseline scan (without regard to timing of baseline scan) – CSF-specific (i.e. not in serum) oligoclonal bands
	CONTINUED ON REVERSE

Colored text= revisions compared to previous McDonald Criteria

KEY: **CIS**: clinically isolated syndrome **CNS**: central nervous system **CSF**: cerebrospinal fluid **DIS**: dissemination in space **DIT**: dissemination in time **T2 lesion**: hyperintense lesion on T2-weighted MRI

*Thompson AJ, et al. Lancet Neurol 2017; online Dec 21. http://dx.doi.org/10.1016/S1474-4422(17)30470-2.

2017 McDonald Criteria for the Diagnosis of Multiple Sclerosis (continued)

CLINICAL PRESENTATION	ADDITIONAL DATA NEEDED TO MAKE MS DIAGNOSIS
...in a person with a typical attack/CIS at onset (continued)	(see KEY on reverse for definitions)
• 1 attack and objective clinical evidence of 1 lesion	**One** of these criteria: – **DIS**: additional attack implicating different CNS site – **DIS**: ≥1 MS-typical symptomatic or asymptomatic T2 lesions in ≥2 areas of CNS: periventricular, juxtacortical/cortical, infratentorial or spinal cord **AND** **One** of these criteria: – **DIT**: additional clinical attack – **DIT**: simultaneous presence of both enhancing and non-enhancing symptomatic or asymptomatic MS-typical MRI lesions – **DIT**: by new T2 or enhancing MRI lesion compared to baseline scan (without regard to timing of baseline scan) – CSF-specific (i.e. not in serum) oligoclonal bands
...in a person with progression of disability from onset	
• progression from onset	– 1 year of disability progression (retrospective or prospective) **AND** **Two** of these criteria: – ≥1 symptomatic or asymptomatic MS-typical T2 lesions (periventricular, juxtacortical/cortical or infratentorial) – ≥2 T2 spinal cord lesions – CSF-specific (i.e. not in serum) oligoclonal bands

The International Panel on Diagnosis of Multiple Sclerosis was convened under the auspices of the International Advisory Committee on Clinical Trials in MS, sponsored by the National MS Society and the European Committee for Treatment and Research in Multiple Sclerosis.

More resources for clinicians: https://www.nationalmssociety.org/For-Professionals/Physicians

Table 2.
McDonald criteria 2017.

5.4 Antiphospholipid antibody syndrome

The antiphospholipid syndrome (APS) is a systemic autoimmune disorder with arterial and venous thromboses; recurrent foetal loss, often accompanied by thrombocytopenia; raised antiphospholipid antibodies, namely, lupus anticoagulant; and anticardiolipin antibodies [39]. Common presentations that can mimic MS are stroke-like presentations such as transient ischemic attack, ischemic stroke, venous thrombosis, epilepsy, headache, movement disorder, transverse myelitis, cognitive impairment, and other neuropsychiatric manifestations.

5.5 Systemic lupus erythematous

Systemic lupus erythematous is an autoimmune condition that is frequency associated with neuropsychiatric manifestations and neurological deficit [13].

MRI characteristics	ADEM: Typical	MS: Typical
Deep gray matter and cortical involvement	Yes	No
Bilateral diffuse lesions	Yes	No
Poorly marginated lesions	Yes	No
Large globular lesions	Yes	No
Periventricular pattern of lesions	No	Yes
Lesions perpendicular to long axis of corpus callosum	No	Yes
Ovoid lesions	No	Yes
Lesions confined to corpus callosum	No	Yes
Sole presence of well-defined lesions	No	Yes
Black holes (on T1 sequence)	No	Yes

Table 3.
Features of MOG antibody disease, NMOSD and MS. (Adapted from [34]).

6. Conclusion

Multiple sclerosis can be challenging to make a diagnosis unless a clinician is familiar with the disease. No better explanation for the condition is essential to come to a conclusion regarding the diagnosis. A good history, elaborate and extensive clinical examination, lumbar puncture, magnetic resonance examination, and blood investigations are required. The McDonald criteria have facilitated the diagnosis of multiple sclerosis for precision and allowing earlier diagnosis.

Author details

Joyce Pauline Joseph
Department of Neurology, Hospital Kuala Lumpur, Malaysia

*Address all correspondence to: jpjmy@yahoo.com

References

[1] Schumacher GA, Beebe G, Kibler RF, Kurland LT, Kurtzke JF, McDowell F, et al. Problems of experimental trials of therapy In multiple sclerosis: Report by the panel on the evaluation of experimental trials of therapy in multiple sclerosis. Annals of the New York Academy of Sciences. 1965;**122**: 552-568

[2] Poser CM, Paty DW, Scheinberg L, et al. New diagnostic criteria for multiple sclerosis: Guidelines for research protocols. Annals of Neurology. Mar 1983;**13**(3):227-231

[3] Polman CH, Reingold SC, Edan G, Filippi M, Hartung H-P, Kappos L, et al. Diagnostic criteria for multiple sclerosis: 2005 revisions to the 'McDonald criteria. Annals of Neurology. 2005;**58**(6): 840-846. CiteSeerX 10.1.1.604.2677. DOI: 10.1002/ana.20703. PMID 16283615

[4] Polman CH, Reingold SC, Banwell B, Clanet M, Cohen JA, Filippi M, et al. Diagnostic criteria for multiple sclerosis: 2010 revisions to the McDonald criteria. Annals of Neurology. 2011;**69**(2): 292-302. DOI: 10.1002/ana.22366. PMC: 3084507. PMID: 21387374

[5] Thompson AJ, Banwell BL, Barkhof F, et al. Diagnosis of multiple sclerosis: 2017 revisions of the McDonald criteria. Lancet Neurology. 2018;**17**(2):162-173

[6] Lublin FD, Reingold SC, Cohen JA, et al. Defining the clinical course of multiple sclerosis: The 2013 revisions. Neurology. 2014;**83**(3):278-286

[7] Balcer LJ. Clinical practice. Optic neuritis. The New England Journal of Medicine. 2006;**354**(12): 1273-1280

[8] Hickman SJ, Dalton CM, Miller DH. Management of acute optic neuritis. Lancet. 2002;**360**:1953-1962

[9] Beck RW, Cleary PA, Anderson MM. A randomized controlled trial of corticosteroids in the treatment of acute optic neuritis. The New England Journal of Medicine. 1992;**326**:581-588

[10] Soderstrom M. Optic neuritis and multiple sclerosis. Acta Ophthalmologica Scandinavica. 2001; **79**:223-227

[11] Optic Neuritis Study Group. The clinical profile of optic neuritis: Experience of the Optic Neuritis Treatment Trial. Archives of Ophthalmology. 1991;**109**:1673-1678

[12] Lee AG, Brazis PW. Clinical Pathways in Neuro-Ophthalmology: An Evidence-Based Approach. New York: Thieme Medical Publishers; 2003

[13] Compston A, McDonald I, Noseworthy J, Lassmann H, Miller D, Smith K, et al. McAlpine's Multiple Sclerosis. 4th ed2005

[14] Swingler RJ, Compston DA. The morbidity of multiple sclerosis. The Quarterly Journal of Medicine. 1992; **83**(300):325-337

[15] Godin D. Multiple Sclerosis and Related Disorders, 3rd Series. Vol. 1222014. Copyright: © Elsevier 2014. eBook ISBN: 9780444633095

[16] Wilkins A. Cerebellar dysfunction in multiple sclerosis. Frontiers in Neurology. 2017;**8**:312. DOI: 10.3389/fneur.2017.00312. Recollection 2017

[17] Alusi SH, Worthington J, Glickman S. Bain PG A study of tremor in multiple sclerosis. Brain. 2001;**124**(Pt. 4):720-730

[18] nationalmssociety.org

[19] McDonald WI, Compston A, Edan G, Goodkin D, Hartung H-P, Lublin FD,

et al. Recommended diagnostic criteria for multiple sclerosis: Guidelines from the international panel on the diagnosis of multiple sclerosis. Annals of Neurology. 2001;**50**(1):121-127

[20] Gastaldi M. Cerebrospinal fluid analysis and the determination of oligoclonal bands. Neurological Sciences. 2017;**38**(Supp. 2): 217-224. DOI: 10.1007/s10072-017-3034-2

[21] Stangel M, Fredrikson S, Meinl E, Petzold A, Stüve O, Tumani H. The utility of cerebrospinal fluid analysis in patients with multiple sclerosis. Nature Reviews. Neurology. 2013;**9**(5):267-276. DOI: 10.1038/nrneurol.2013.41. Epub 2013 Mar 26

[22] Davenport RD, Keren DF. Oligoclonal bands in cerebrospinal fluids: Significance of corresponding bands in serum for diagnosis of multiple sclerosis. Clinical Chemistry. 1988; **34**(4):764-765

[23] Walsh P, Kane N, Butler S. The clinical role of evoked potentials. Journal of Neurology, Neurosurgery, and Psychiatry. 2005 Jun;**76**(Supp. 2): ii16-ii22

[24] Traboulsee A, Simon JH, Stone L, et al. Revised recommendations of the consortium of MS centers task force for a standardized MRI protocol and clinical guidelines for the diagnosis and follow-up of multiple sclerosis. AJNR. American Journal of Neuroradiology. 2016;**37**(3):394-401

[25] Consortium of MS Centers MRI Protocol and Clinical Guidelines for the Diagnosis and Follow-up of MS. 2018. REVISED GUIDELINES. www.mscare.org/mri

[26] Huang D, Swanson EA, Lin CP, Schuman JS, Stinson WG, Chang W, et al. Optical coherence tomography. Science. 1991;**254**(5035):1178-1181

[27] Britze J, Frederiksen JL. Optical coherence tomography in multiple sclerosis. Eye (Lond). 2018;**32**:884-888. DOI: 10.1038/s41433-017-0010-2

[28] Lennon VA, Wingerchuk DM, Kryzer TJ, et al. A serum autoantibody marker of neuromyelitis optica: Distinction from multiple sclerosis. Lancet. 2004;**364**:2106-2112

[29] Lennon VA, Kryzer TJ, Pittock SJ, Verkman AS, Hinson SR. IgG marker of optic-spinal multiple sclerosis binds to the aquaporin-4 water channel. The Journal of Experimental Medicine. 2005; **202**:473-477

[30] Wingerchuk DM, Banwell B, Bennett JL, Cabre P, Carroll W, Chitnis T, et al. International consensus diagnostic criteria for neuromyelitis optica spectrum disorders. Neurology. 2015;**85**(2):177-189. DOI: 10.1212/WNL.0000000000001729. Epub 2015 Jun 19

[31] Johns TG, Bernard CC. The structure and function of myelin oligodendrocyte glycoprotein. Journal of Neurochemistry. 1999;**72**(1):1-9

[32] Baumann M, Sahin K, Lechner C, et al. Clinical and neuroradiological differences of paediatric acute disseminating encephalomyelitis with and without antibodies to the myelin oligodendrocyte glycoprotein. Journal of Neurology, Neurosurgery, and Psychiatry. 2015;**86**:265-272

[33] Zhou D, Srivastava R, Nessler S, et al. Identification of a pathogenic antibody response to native myelin oligodendrocyte glycoprotein in multiple sclerosis. Proceedings of the National Academy of Sciences of the United States of America. 2006;**103**:19057-19062. [PMC free article] [PubMed]

[34] Jarius S, Ruprecht K, Kleiter I, Borisow N, Asgari N, Pitarokoili K, et al. MOG-IgG in NMO and related

disorders: A multicenter study of 50 patients. Part 2: Epidemiology, clinical presentation, radiological and laboratory features, treatment responses, and long-term outcome. Journal of Neuroinflammation. 2016; **13**(1):280

[35] Pohl D, Alper G, Van Haren K, Kornberg AJ, Lucchinetti CF, Tenembaum S, et al. Acute disseminated encephalomyelitis updates on an inflammatory CNS syndrome. Neurology. 2016;**87**(Supp. 2):S38-45

[36] Garg RK. Acute disseminated encephalomyelitis. Postgraduate Medical Journal. 2003;**79**:11-17

[37] Krupp LB, Banwell B, Tenembaum S, International Pediatric MS Study Group. Consensus definitions proposed for pediatric multiple sclerosis and related disorders. Neurology. 2007;**68** (16, supplement 2):S7-S12

[38] Krupp LB, Tardieu M, Amato MP, et al. International pediatric multiple sclerosis study group criteria for pediatric multiple sclerosis and immune-mediated central nervous system demyelinating disorders: Revisions to the 2007 definitions. Multiple Sclerosis Journal. 2013;**19**(10): 1261-1267

[39] Asherson RA, Cervera R, Piette JC, Shoenfeld Y. The antiphospholipid syndrome: History, definition, classification, and differential diagnosis. In: Asherson RA, Cervera R, Piette JC, Shoenfeld Y, editors. The Antiphospholipid Syndrome. Boca Raton (FL): CRC Press; 1996. pp. 3-12

Section 4

Mental Decline in MS

Chapter 4

Neuropsychological Functions and Cognitive Neurorehabilitation in Multiple Sclerosis

Lambros Messinis, Grigorios Nasios and Panagiotis Papathanasopouos

Abstract

Although cognitive difficulties are not frequently reported by patients among the initial symptoms of Multiple Sclerosis (MS), there is sufficient evidence that cognitive impairment is present from the early stage of the disease. Today it is commonly accepted that roughly one-half of individuals with MS will experience cognitive dysfunction over the course of the disease. Though MS was originally considered a disease of white matter, more recent investigations with advanced immunohistochemistry techniques have revealed that demyelination of gray matter is a common neuropathological feature in MS contributing significantly to cognitive impairment. However, despite now been recognized as a core symptom of MS, evidence up till now is only modest regarding the efficacy of pharmacological agents on cognitive dysfunction and non-pharmacological interventions such as cognitive rehabilitation also provide incomplete evidence on whether they might improve or stabilize cognitive impairment and especially over long follow up periods. Despite this general consensus, there are studies that have reported the efficacy of cognitive neurorehabilitation in reducing MS associated cognitive deficits. In this chapter we provide a selective review of the most relevant features related to this topic.

Keywords: multiple sclerosis, neuropsychological functions, cognition, cognitive neurorehabilitation

1. Introduction

Historically the disease today known as multiple sclerosis (MS) has been referred to in the historical medical literature with a variety of terms, including, disseminated sclerosis and sclerose en plaque [1]. Lidwina van Schiedam, was the first potential case of MS dating as far back as 1421, when Jan van Berieren commented on her illness. Records showed that she had difficulties walking, paralysis of the right arm, decreased sensation and visual difficulties [2].

Today we know that MS is a chronic inflammatory autoimmune degenerative disease of the central nervous system (CNS). It is the most common non-traumatic neurological disorder among young adults leading to disability. The etiology of MS involves white matter pathology, cortical atrophy, cortical lesions, and microstructural abnormalities in deep gray matter that impact structural and functional connectivity [3]. Cognitive impairment in MS appears to be a result of this diffuse disruption in brain networks [4]. These patients may also present sensorimotor [5], visual [6], bladder, cerebellar [7] and emotional difficulties leading to functional disability [8] and poorer quality of life [9].

Environmental factors and especially geographical latitude may significantly influence the development of MS. However, genetic susceptibility as is evident from twin studies and familial cases, suggests that MS disease causality is due to a complex interaction between multiple genes and environmental factors, eventually leading to inflammatory-mediated central nervous system deterioration [10]. Genomic studies, with specific HLA antigens (HLA-DR2), have confirmed the genetic susceptibility of MS [10]. Numerous other environmental factors have been evaluated that may be associated with MS, but methodological caveats have casted doubts on their validity. On average, MS patients contracted common childhood illnesses at later ages than healthy controls [11]. A biomarker of Epstein-Barr virus (anti-EBNA IgG seropositivity), infectious mononucleosis, and smoking have shown the strongest consistent evidence of an association. However, additional data and better-designed studies are needed to establish robust evidence [12].

MS disease course is heterogeneous in nature and several types have been described: Relapsing remitting MS (RRMS), Active (with relapses and/or new lesions on MRI), Not Active (no relapses or MRI activity), Progressive MS (Secondary Progressive MS (SPMS) and Primary Progressive MS (PPMS), Active with Progression (relapses/MRI activity and clinical deterioration not due to relapses), Active but without Progression (relapses but no clinical deterioration), Not Active but with Progression, Not Active and without Progression (stable disease) [13]. The use of these terms is primarily for descriptive purposes and for setting reasonable expectations for treatment.

This chapter is not a comprehensive review of the extensive literature on neuropsychological functions and cognitive rehabilitation in multiple sclerosis, but rather a selective review of the most relevant features related to this topic.

2. Neuropsychological functions in multiple sclerosis

Dating back to the seminal writings on MS, Charcot's observations of the adverse effects that MS exerts on memory, concept formation, and the intellect [14], were underestimated for many decades in the neurology literature. It was only with the emergence of the comprehensive care model in the early 1980s, that the nature and significance of cognitive dysfunction in MS became appreciated. The medical community, due to the often-subtle nature of cognitive deficits in MS, and the difficulty in detecting these deficits during routine clinical practice, was initially slow to appreciate them as a core clinical symptom of MS. Instead, they believed that cognitive impairment was a relatively rare entity in MS, occurred only in advanced cases with a high level of physical disability and was associated with subcortical dementia [15].

Cognitive difficulties are not frequently reported by patients among the initial symptoms of MS, although there is sufficient evidence that cognitive impairment is present from the early stage of the disease (see for e.g., the study by [16], which assessed MS patients neuropsychologically, not more than 2 years after experiencing their first neurological symptoms, and [17], who presents three cases evaluated at different stages of the disease). Moreover, cognitive impairment may be present in the early stages of the disease in patients with relatively low or mild physical disability (see for e.g. the studies by [18, 19] who found cognitive deficits in patients with an EDSS disability score of ≤ 3.5, that had not yet been influenced significantly in their daily functional abilities and employment status). A recent anatomofunctional study utilizing diffusion imaging and resting state functional MRI, revealed that disconnection in the default mode network (DMN) and attentional networks (ATT), may deprive the brain of the necessary compensatory mechanisms required to face the widespread structural damage during the early course of MS, providing a possible explanation for the cognitive dysfunction in these early stages of the disease [20].

Although it is now commonly accepted that roughly one-half of individuals with MS [21, 22], will experience clinical deficits over the course of the disease, prevalence rates are highly variable and depend to a large extent on the type of MS population studied, the clinical, demographic and sociodemographic characteristics and the year conducted. A recent study that included RRMS and SPMS patients attending an outpatient neurology clinic reported an overall cognitive dysfunction prevalence rate of 53.7% [23]. Moreover, the study by [22], reported that 47% of their MS patients recruited from an outpatient clinical setting, diagnosed with the revised McDonald criteria [24], the majority with RRMS and mean duration of illness at 9.6 years, assessed with a brief cognitive measure (BICAMS), performed below the 1SD cutoff set for impairment on at least one of the three tests that comprise this brief neuropsychological battery. In an interesting cross-sectional study that evaluated the patterns of cognitive impairment in patients with disease duration of up to 30 years, 20.9% performed below the 1SD cutoff for impairment by the 5th year from disease onset, by 10 years this had reached 29.3%. By utilizing regression modeling the authors suggested that cognitive impairment may precede MS onset by 1.2 years [25].

Most of the evidence suggests that cognitive impairment in MS patients is present during all disease stages and across all disease clinical subtypes [26–28], including, RRMS, PPMS, SPMS, Clinically Isolated Syndrome (CIS) and "benign MS" [29, 30], and even Radiologically Isolated Syndrome—(RIS) [31]. Based on the majority of studies that have compared cognitive functions across disease subtype, deficits appear to be more frequent and more widespread in the progressive type rather than in the relapsing form of the disease [23, 29, 31–32].

The dissemination of lesions in cerebral white matter including their affinity for periventricular regions provides the basis for some cognitive dysfunction commonalities [33]. In this respect, some cognitive domains appear to be more commonly compromised than others. Information processing efficiency, episodic memory, attention, and executive functioning are the domains found predominantly to be detrimentally affected in MS [21, 34, 35]. Among these domains the most common pattern involves circumscribed deficits as a combination of one or two of the above-mentioned domains (e.g., attention/processing speed, learning/memory, and or executive functions [11, 15, 21].

Symptoms like cognitive and physical fatigue, which are often accompanied by depression and anxiety, may negatively influence cognition in MS patients. This is especially true when extended periods are required to complete and appear more relevant for the patient's daily life than what may be assumed by many physicians treating MS patients [11].

Although cognitive impairment is highly prevalent among MS patients, some have a tendency to withstand severe disease burden (e.g., white matter lesions and cerebral atrophy), and present with overall lower levels of cognitive decline. One possible explanation for this protective mechanism is the brain reserve hypothesis and the cognitive reserve theory [36]. Recently, it has been verified that highly significant protection for cognitive impairment is provided by brain reserve, defined as the maximal lifetime brain growth (MLBG), and estimated with intracranial volume or head circumference. Larger MLBG a proxy for neuronal and synaptic count has been linked to lower risk for cognitive impairment in MS [37]. This larger MLBG appears to be associated with more robust neural networks resistant to disease-related disruption and also provides more potential degrees of freedom for the brain to plastically reorganize in the face of MS disease related challenges.

2.1 Assessment of neuropsychological functions in MS

The multidimensional nature of cognitive dysfunction in MS necessitates an assessment of numerous cognitive domains. The challenge until recently was to find the optimal combination of cognitive tests that would provide an accurate picture of the deficits whilst avoiding the use of unnecessary and time-consuming measures [15].

In order to overcome some of the limitations in assessing cognition in MS, and considering the fact that not all neuropsychological measures are appropriate for the MS population, a number of neuropsychological assessment tools (brief screening batteries and comprehensive neuropsychological batteries), have been utilized specifically for this population in routine clinical care and for research purposes. **Table 1** provides a summary of the most important neuropsychological tools utilized in MS patients.

2.2 Neuropsychological functions and neuroimaging

Although MS was originally considered to be a disease of White Matter (WM), more recently with the development and utilization of advanced immunohisto-chemistry techniques investigators have begun to appreciate that demyelination of gray matter (GM) is a common neuropathological feature in MS patients. Demyelination of GM appears to be more common in the cerebellum, spinal cord and hippocampus. Essentially, however, no areas within the CNS are actually spared [38]. The thalamus is considered the most frequently affected subcortical

Cognitive domain	Rao brief repeatable neuropsychological battery (BRB)	Minimal assessment of cognitive function in MS (MACFIMS)	NINDS common data elements	Brief assessment of multiple sclerosis (BICAMS)
Cognitive processing speed	SDMT	SDMT	SDMT	SDMT
	PASAT	PASAT	PASAT	—
Language	COWAT	COWAT	COWAT	—
Visual/ spatial	—	JLO	—	—
Memory	SRT	CVLT2	CVLT2	CVLT2
	10/36 Spatial Recall Test	BVMTR	BVMTR	BVMTR
Executive function	—	D-KEFS	D-KEFS	—

SDMT: Symbol Digits Modalities Test; PASAT: Paced Auditory Serial Addition Test; COWAT: Controlled Oral Word Association Test; CVLT2: California Verbal Learning Test 2nd edition; BVMTR: Brief Visuospatial Memory Test Revised; DKEFS: Delis Kaplan Executive Function System Sorting Test.

Table 1.
Neuropsychological batteries utilized in MS patients.

GM structure, but lesions have been identified within the putamen, pallidum, caudate, amygdale, substantia nigra and hypothalamus [39].

Considering the above, clinicians and researchers investigating neuropsychological functions in MS patients have realized that cognitive dysfunction in this population cannot be explained by WM pathology alone. GM pathology appears to have a significant impact on cognitive impairment, but requires novel neuroimaging technology in order to detect and visualize these types of lesions. Due to these visualization difficulties in current imaging technologies, research in MS has shifted its focus primarily to comparing WM and GM measures of atrophy [39]. In this respect, [40], noted a similar increase in WM atrophy across disease stages (three-fold), whereas, atrophy of the GM increased proportionally according to disease stage, i.e. three-fold in CIS converting to RRMS, versus 14-fold in SPMS patients.

Another important issue is that GM atrophy has been reported to be regionally specific, involving early volume loss of the basal ganglia, corpus callosum and thalamus. Recent studies have outlined the significance of thalamic volume in relation to cognitive impairment. One such report by [41] found lower thalamic volumes in MS patients compared to healthy participants, with the lowest volumes found in severely cognitive impaired patients. In one of our recent studies, we provide evidence that thalamic atrophy was the best predictor of cognitive dysfunction in RRMS patients and was also highly associated with activities of daily living and employment status [42]. Moreover, in a similar study that recruited late stage SPMS patients, we found that corpus callosum atrophy was associated with deficits in cognitive flexibility, processing speed, episodic memory, executive functions, reaction time and phonological verbal fluency. Processing speed and composite memory were the most sensitive markers for predicting employment status. Corpus callosum atrophy was the most sensitive MRI marker for episodic memory and processing speed deficits. Moreover, corpus callosum atrophy predicted a clinically meaningful cognitive decline, affecting employment status in our SPMS patients [43]. Thus, it appears that irreversible tissue loss, as measured by brain atrophy of the white and gray matter, is strongly associated to cognitive function in the MS population. While white matter atrophy has also been reported to contribute significantly to impairment in mental processing speed and working memory, gray matter atrophy was highly predictive for verbal memory status, but additionally predicted neuropsychiatric symptoms such as disinhibition and euphoria [44].

3. Interventions for cognitive dysfunction in multiple sclerosis

Recent evidence from empirical research has indicated that cognitive dysfunction in MS patients is highly related to everyday functioning abilities [45]. One such study that evaluated associations between cognitive functions and objective performance on measures of everyday functioning in MS, [46], reported that MS patients had significantly more difficulties in simple and more complex cooking abilities, using the phone, taking medication, and paying the bills, compared to healthy participants. An interesting study by O'Brien et al. [47] and a more ecologically valid study by Goverover et al [48], utilizing an actual reality (AR) approach through the use of everyday tasks requiring the internet (e.g. booking an airline ticket, purchasing cookies and ordering pizza), the authors report significant correlations between these tasks and performance on mental processing speed (SDMT), concluding that this measure contributes significantly to predicting everyday functioning capacity in MS. A more recent study, [48], examined the ability of MS patients to manage their finances. The authors found that MS patients demonstrated and reported more difficulties in managing their finances compared to healthy controls. Moreover, MS patient's difficulties in handling their finances were associated with the severity of cognitive dysfunction. As this important everyday task requires intact mental processing ability and executive-attentional abilities, domains usually impaired in MS individuals, these findings may serve as potential intervention indicators when planning cognitive rehabilitation interventions.

From the findings reported by the studies mentioned previously, it becomes obvious that interventions to alleviate, stabilize, reduce or compensate for cognitive impairment are of an extremely high priority, in order to provide MS individuals with the necessary mechanisms to better handle their everyday functioning disabilities. The evidence up till now is only modest regarding the efficacy of pharmacological agents on cognitive dysfunction [49, 50], and non-pharmacological interventions such as cognitive rehabilitation also provide incomplete evidence on whether they might improve or stabilize cognitive impairment and especially over long follow up periods [51]. Despite this general consensus, there are studies that have reported the efficacy of pharmacological agents [52] and cognitive rehabilitation [28, 53, 54] in reducing MS associated cognitive deficits.

3.1 Cognitive neurorehabilitation in multiple sclerosis

The goals of non-pharmacological treatments for MS-related cognitive deficits are similar to those of the immune-modulating drugs. In other words, these interventions are used with the intent of preventing the progression of cognitive dysfunction and promoting a therapeutic 'milieu' in which optimal cognitive functioning can occur, and include specific approaches which are known to be effective in remediating cognitive disorders of any etiology [15]. Cognitive rehabilitation or 'rehabilitation of individuals with cognitive impairment' [55] include specific approaches designed to assist the MS patient to better cope with existing cognitive impairments or to improve a specific cognitive skill. It focuses on two main approaches: the restorative or functional training approach (i.e. ameliorating patients' deficits in processing and interpreting information—e.g. when cognitive training is used to enhance attention or memory performance). The restorative approach depends on the brains capability of cortical reorganization following injury (i.e. that the brain possesses some degree of plasticity). The second is the compensatory or strategy training approach (e.g. modifying the patient's environment, using a calendar and set phone reminders). These approaches have different goals and limitations, and may be used in isolation or in combination. For example, in patients with extensive tissue loss, neural plasticity might be hampered and no or little effect will result from restorative or functional training. In that particular patient, compensatory or strategy training might help the patient to work around the problems that are present. As for most MS patients, especially those with a relapsing disease course, it is expected that restorative or functional training will lead to improved cognitive functioning on neuropsychological measures, improved functioning in everyday life activities, and ultimately will lead to an improvement in network efficiency [56].

Several studies have investigated the effectiveness of cognitive rehabilitation interventions in patients with MS, including computer-based training and neuropsychological counseling, but with inconsistent results. The majority of studies found improvements in specific cognitive domains, but the evidence provided in the literature remains inconclusive [57]. A significant limitation in providing evidence on the efficacy of studies involving cognitive rehabilitation is the great variability in the methods or strategies utilized for treatment, the measures used to assess cognition and other secondary outcome variables and the lack of ecologically valid outcome measures in order to assess the efficiency of these interventions in everyday functioning ability.

Applying a technique known as the Story Memory Technique (SMT), [58] provided class 1 evidence that this technique applied for 5 weeks/twice weekly (10 sessions) with an emphasis on teaching context and imagery to facilitate learning, improved episodic memory in MS patients relative to controls and moreover produced increased f-MRI activation during a memory task in frontal and parietal regions. Positive effects were additionally observed for objective measures of everyday memory function, general contentment, and executive functioning. These positive outcomes were sustained for a period of 6 months.

Clinical trials utilizing the RehaCom computerized software in MS patients with cognitive impairments have also shown positive outcomes. Bonavita et al. [59], noted significant pre-to post treatment improvements in a RehaCom treated MS cohort, on mental information processing, executive functions and attention. This and other similar studies have reported positive outcomes in MS patients treated with this software, and moreover, associations between functional neuroimaging (f-MRI) findings with changes in neurocognitive measures have been reported [59–61]. In a multicenter Italian study, RehaCom was utilized to provide specific intensive cognitive training for 12 months. Results showed that MS patients treated with this modality had improved scores post treatment on the SDMT, PASAT, and episodic memory measures relative to MS patients who received aspecific psychological therapy for the same period of time [62].

In 2017, our group, [53], conducted a multicenter randomized controlled trial with 58 clinically stable RRMS patients utilizing computer-assisted (RehaCom) functional cognitive training with an emphasis on episodic memory, information processing speed/attention, and executive functions for 10 weeks. Our findings revealed that only the group that had received functional cognitive training showed significant improvements in verbal and visuospatial episodic memory, processing speed/attention, and executive functioning from pre—to postassessment. Moreover, the improvement obtained on attention was retained over 6 months providing evidence on the long term benefits of this intervention. Treated patients rated the intervention positively and were more confident about their cognitive abilities following treatment.

While the previously mentioned positive results regarding the efficacy of cognitive rehabilitation interventions in MS individuals cannot be overstated, it is important to note that a recently published Cochrane Review that included 15 studies and 989 MS participants regarding the efficacy of memory retraining techniques with or without the assistance of computer software, concluded that there is only limited evidence on the effectiveness of memory rehabilitation in this population. The authors further suggest that more RCTs of high methodological quality be conducted with the utilization of ecologically valid outcome assessments [63].

Another Cochrane Review that included 20 studies and 966 MS participants evaluating the effectiveness of neuropsychological rehabilitation in MS [64], reported low-level evidence for the positive effects of neuropsychological rehabilitation in this population. However, the authors reported that the comparability of the 20 studies reviewed was limited due to heterogeneity of interventions and outcome measures. It should be noted however, that the majority of studies included in this review did show some evidence of positive effects on cognitive outcome measures.

Despite the limitations noted by the previously mentioned Cochrane reviews, a growing body of literature supports the efficacy of cognitive rehabilitation for individuals with MS and more randomized controlled trials are needed to support existing and new rehabilitation techniques. Cognitive rehabilitation appears to be useful for all patients with MS regardless of disease course and level of cognitive impairment, although studies including exclusively MS patients with progressive disease course are limited. Future clinical trials utilizing cognitive rehabilitation interventions in progressive MS patients should become a priority.

4. Conclusions

Cognitive impairment is frequently encountered in MS individuals, irrespective of disease duration, severity of physical disability, and at both the earlier and later disease stages. Moreover, cognitive dysfunction in this population may have a significant negative impact on quality of life, activities of daily living and employment status. Furthermore, past and current pharmacological treatments have shown inconsistent findings in alleviating cognitive impairment in individuals with MS requiring further clarification. This inconsistency regarding the effects of pharmacological interventions on cognition, coupled with the reduced ability to effectively handle everyday tasks, loss of employment and social interaction capacity, prioritizes the need for utilizing potentially more effective non-pharmacological, neurobehavioral interventions to address cognitive dysfunction and everyday functioning abilities. Neurobehavioral interventions utilizing cognitive rehabilitation have shown favorable effects on MS patients cognitive performance and other related skills, and in some cases, have managed to generalize these positive effects to MS individual's everyday life functioning ability. In this respect it becomes obvious that there is a need for rigorous new cognitive neurorehabilitation studies that may overcome some of the methodological limitations of older studies, and provide robust evidence regarding the efficiency of such cognitive interventions for the MS population.

Conflict of interest

The authors have no conflict of interest.

Declarations

Parts of this chapter originate from my Doctoral Dissertation entitled: Neuropsychological functions and association with Single Photon Emission Computed Tomography (SPECT) in Greek Multiple Sclerosis patients: Efficacy of a Computerized Cognitive Rehabilitation Intervention (2017). Department of Neurology, University of Patras Medical School, Patras, Greece.

Author details

Lambros Messinis[1*], Grigorios Nasios[2] and Panagiotis Papathanasopouos[3]

1 Neuropsychology Section, Departments of Psychiatry and Neurology, University Hospital of Patras and University of Patras Medical School, Greece

2 Department of Speech and Language Therapy, School of Health Sciences, University of Ioannina, Greece

3 University of Patras Medical School, Greece

*Address all correspondence to: lmessinis@upatras.gr

References

[1] Murray TJ. The history of multiple sclerosis. In: Burks JS, Johnson KP, editors. Multiple Sclerosis: Diagnosis, Medical Management and Rehabilitation. New York: Demos Medical Publishing Murray; 2000

[2] Kesselring J. History of multiple sclerosis. In: Raine CS, McFarland HF, Hohlfeld R, editors. Multiple Sclerosis: A Comprchensive Text. Philadelphia, PA: Elsevier Limited. Kesselring; 2008

[3] Massimiliano DF, Portaccio E, Mancini A, et al. Multiple sclerosis and cognition: Synaptic failure and network dysfunction. Nature Reviews. Neuroscience. 2018;**19**:599-609

[4] Schoonheim MM, Meijer KA, Geurts JJ. Network collapse and cognitive impairment in multiple sclerosis. Frontiers in Neurology. 2015;**6**:82-86

[5] Peterson DS, Fling BW. How changes in brain activity and connectivity are associated with motor performance in people with MS. NeuroImage: Clinical. 2018;**17**:153-162

[6] Balcer LJ, Balk LJ, Brandt AU, et al. The international multiple sclerosis visual system consortium: Advancing visual system research in multiple sclerosis. Journal of Neuro-Ophthalmology. 2018;**38**:494-501

[7] Doty RL, MacGillivray MR, Talab H, et al. Balance in multiple sclerosis: Relationship to central brain regions. Experimental Brain Research. 2018;**236**: 2739-2750

[8] Uitdehaag BM. Disability outcome measures in phase III clinical trials in multiple sclerosis. CNS Drugs. 2018;**1**: 1-16

[9] Kefaliakos A, Pliakos I, Diomidous M. Managing the quality of life in patients with multiple sclerosis: A literature review. Studies in Health Technology and Informatics. 2016;**226**: 220-221

[10] Hawkes CH, Macgregor AJ. Twin studies and the heritability of MS: A conclusion. Multiple Sclerosis. 2009;**15**: 661-667

[11] Lezak MD, Howieson DB, Bigler ED, Tranel D. Neuropsychological Assessment. 5th ed. New York: Oxford University Press; 2012. pp. 290-303

[12] Belbasis L, Bellou V, Evangelou E, Ioannidis JPA, Tzoulaki I. Environmental risk actors and multiple sclerosis: An umbrella review of systematic reviews and meta-analyses. Lancet Neurology. 2015;**14**:263-273

[13] Lublin FD, Reingold SC, Cohen JA, et al. Defining the clinical course of multiple sclerosis: The 2013 revisions. Neurology. 2014;**83**:278-286

[14] Charcot JM. Lectures on the Diseases of the Nervous System. London: New Sydenham Society; 1877

[15] Messinis L, Kosmidis MH, Lyros E, Papathanasopoulos P. Assessment and rehabilitation of cognitive impairment in multiple sclerosis. International Review of Psychiatry. 2010;**22**:22-34

[16] Schulz D, Kopp B, Kunkel A, Faiss JH. Cognition in the early stage of multiple sclerosis. Journal of Neurology. 2006;**253**:1002-1010

[17] Faiss JH. Cognitive dysfunction in different stages in multiple sclerosis—presentation of 3 cases. Journal of Neurology. 2007;**254**(supp. 2):77-79

[18] Ruggieri RM, Palermo R, Vitello G, Gennuso M, Settipani N, Picolli F. Cognitive impairment in patients suffering from relapsing-remitting multiple sclerosis with EDSS ≤ 3.5. Acta

Neurologica Scandinavica. 2003;**108**: 323-326

[19] Messinis L, Anyfantis E, Paschali A, Papathanasopoulos P. Cognitive deficits in relapsing remitting multiple sclerosis patients with low disability status. In: Proceedings of the 7th International Congress on the Improvement of the Quality of life on Dementia, Parkinson's disease, Epilepsy, MS, Muscular Disorders and Neuroethics. 2009. pp. 31-35

[20] Louapre C, Perlbarg V. Garcia-Lorenzo, et al., Brain networks disconnection in early multiple sclerosis: An anatomofunctional study. Human Brain Mapping. 2014;**35**:4706-4717

[21] Chiaravalloti ND, DeLuca J. Cognitive impairment in multiple sclerosis. Lancet Neurology. 2008;**7**: 1139-1151

[22] Polychroniadou E, Bakirtzis C, Langdon D, et al. Validation of the Brief International Cognitive Assessment for Multiple Sclerosis (BICAMS) in Greek population with multiple sclerosis. Multiple Sclerosis and Related Disorders. 2016;**9**:68-72

[23] Papathanasiou A, Messinis L, Georgiou LV, Papathanasopoulos P. Cognitive impairment in relapsing remitting and secondary progressive multiple sclerosis patients: Efficacy of a computerized cognitive screening battery. ISRN Neurology. 2014;**2014**: 151379. DOI: 10.1155/2014/151379

[24] Polman CH, Reingold SC, Banwell B, et al. Diagnostic criteria for multiple sclerosis: 2010 revisions to the McDonald criteria. Annals of Neurology. 2011;**69**:292-302

[25] Achiron A, Chapman J, Magalashvili D, et al. Modeling of cognitive impairment by disease duration in multiple sclerosis: A cross–sectional study. PLoS One. 2013;**8**(8):e71058

[26] Prakash RS, Snook EM, Lewis JM, et al. Cognitive impairments in relapsing remitting multiple sclerosis: A meta-analysis. Multiple Sclerosis. 2008;**14**: 1250-1261

[27] Langdon DW. Cognition in multiple sclerosis. Current Opinion in Neurology. 2011;**24**:244-249

[28] Rosti-Otajarvi E, Ruutianen J, Huhtala H, Hamalainen P. Cognitive performance profile in different phenotypes of MS with cognitive complaints. Multiple Sclerosis and Related Disorders. 2014;**3**:463-472

[29] Potagas C, Giogkaraki E, Koutsis G, Mandellos D, Tsirempolou E, Sfagos C, et al. Cognitive impairment in different MS subtypes and clinically isolated syndromes. Journal of the Neurological Sciences. 2008;**267**:100-106

[30] Panou T, Mastorodemos V, Papadaki E, Simos PG, Plaitakis A. Early signs of memory impairment among multiple sclerosis patients with clinically isolated syndrome. Behavioural Neurology. 2012;**25**:311-326

[31] Forslin Y, Granberg T, Jumah AA, et al. Incidence of radiologically isolated syndrome: A population-based study. American Journal of Neuroradiology. 2016;**37**:1017-1022

[32] Ntoskou A, Messinis L, Nasios G, Martzoukou M, Makris G, Panagiotopoulos E, et al. Cognitive and language deficits in multiple sclerosis: Comparison of relapsing remitting and secondary progressive subtypes. The Open Neurology Journal. 2018;**12**:19-30

[33] Fischer JS. Cognitive impairments in multiple. In: Cook SD, editor. Handbook of Multiple Sclerosis. New York, USA: Marcel Dekker; 2001. pp. 233-256

[34] Rao SM, Leo GJ, Bernardin L, Unverzagt F. Cognitive dysfunction in multiple sclerosis: I Frequency, patterns,

and prediction. Neurology. 1991;**41**: 685-691

[35] Guimares J, Jose SA. Cognitive dysfunction in multiple sclerosis. Frontiers in Neurology. 2012;**3**:74

[36] Sumowski JF, Leavitt VM. Cognitive reserve in multiple sclerosis. Multiple Sclerosis. 2013;**19**:1122-1127

[37] Sumowski JF, Rocca MA, Leavitt VM, et al. Brain reserve and cognitive reserve protect against cognitive decline over 4.5 years in MS. Neurology. 2014; **82**:1776-1178

[38] Gilmore CP, DeLuca GC, Bo L, et al. Spinal cord neuronal pathology in multiple sclerosis. Brain Pathology. 2009;**19**:642-649

[39] Benedict RHB, DeLuca J, Enzinger C, Geuts JG, Krupp LB, Rao M. Neuropsychology of multiple sclerosis: Looking back and moving forward. Journal of the International Neuropsychological Society. 2017;**23**: 832-842

[40] Fisher E, Lee JC, Nakamura K, Rudick RA. Gray matter atrophy in multiple sclerosis: A longitudinal study. Annals of Neurology. 2008;**64**:255-265

[41] Schoonheim MM, Hulst HE, Brandt RB, et al. Thalamus structure and function determine severity of cognitive impairment in multiple sclerosis. Neurology. 2015;**84**:776-783

[42] Papathanasiou A, Messinis L, Zampakis P, et al. Thalamic atrophy predicts cognitive impairment in relapsing remitting multiple sclerosis. Effect on instrumental activities of daily living and employment status. Journal of the Neurological Sciences. 2015;**358**: 236-242

[43] Papathanasiou A, Messinis L, Zampakis P, Papathanasopoulos P. (2017). Corpus Callosum atrophy as a marker of clinically meaningful cognitive decline in Secondary Progressive multiple sclerosis. Impact on employment status. Journal of Clinical Neuroscience. 2017;**43**:170-175

[44] Lanz M, Hahn HK, Hildebrandt H. Brain atrophy and cognitive impairment in multiple sclerosis: a review. Journal of Neurology. 2007;**254**(Supp. 2):II/43-II/48

[45] Goverover Y, Chiaravalloti N, DeLuca J. Brief international cognitive assessment for multiple sclerosis (BICAMS) and performance of everyday life tasks: Actual reality. Multiple Sclerosis. 2016;**22**:544-550

[46] Goverover Y, Kalmar J, Gaudino-Goering E, et al. The relation between subjective and objective measures of everyday life activities in persons with multiple sclerosis. Archives of Physical Medicine and Rehabilitation. 2005;**86**: 2303-2308

[47] O'Brien A, Gaudino-Goering E, Shawaryn M, Komaroff E, Moore NB, DeLuca J. (2007). Relationship of multiple sclerosis neuropsychological questionnaire (MSNQ) to functional, emotional, and neuropsychological outcomes. Archives of Clinical Neuropsychology. 2007;**22**:933-948

[48] Goverover Y. Cognition and everyday functional activity in persons with multiple sclerosis. In: Presented at the 5th Conference of the International MS Cognition Society. 2016

[49] Roy S, Benedict RH, Drake AS, Weinstock-Guttman B. Impact of pharmacotherapy on cognitive dysfunction in patients with multiple sclerosis. CNS Drugs. 2016;**30**(3): 209-225. DOI: 10.1007/s40263-016-0319-6

[50] Miller E, Morel A, Miller I, Saluk J. Pharmacological treatment and non-pharmacological therapies of cognitive impairment in multiple sclerosis.

Current Neuropharmacology. 2018;**16**: 475-483

[51] Mitolo M, Venneri A, Wilkinson ID, Sharrack B. Cognitive rehabilitation in multiple sclerosis: A systematic review. Journal of Neurological Sciences. 2015; **354**:1-9

[52] Mokhber N, Azarpazhooh A, Orouji E. Cognitive dysfunction in patients with multiple sclerosis treated with different types of interferon beta: A randomized clinical trial. Journal of the Neurological Sciences. 2014;**342**:16-20

[53] Messinis L, Nasios G, Kosmidis MH, Zampakis P, Malefaki S, Ntoskou, et al. Efficacy of a computer—assisted cognitive rehabilitation intervention in relapsing remitting multiple sclerosis patients—a randomized controlled trial. Behavioural Neurology. 2017;**2017**: 5919841

[54] Dardiotis E, Nousia A, Siokas V, Tsouris Z, Andravizou A, Fotios A, et al. Efficacy of computer-based cognitive training in neuropsychological performance of patients with multiple sclerosis: A systematic review and meta-analysis. Multiple Sclerosis and Related Disorders. 2018;**20**:58-66

[55] Sohlberg MM, Mateer CA. Cognitive Rehabilitation: An Integrative Neuropsychological Approach. New York: Guilford Press; 2001

[56] Hulst HE, Langdon DW. Functional training is a senseless strategy in MS cognitive rehabilitation: Strategy training is the only useful approach—NO. Multiple Sclerosis. 2017;**23**:930-932

[57] Bakirtzis C, Ioannidis P, Messinis L, Nasios G, Grigoriadis N. (2018). The rationale for monitoring cognitive function in multiple sclerosis: practical issues for clinicians. The Open Neurology Journal. 2018;**12**:31-40

[58] Chiaravalloti ND, Moore NB, Nikelshpur OM, DeLuca J. An RCT to treat learning impairment in multiple sclerosis. Neurology. 2013;**81**:2066-2072

[59] Bonavita S, Sacco R, Della Corte M, et al. Computer-aided cognitive rehabilitation improves cognitive performances and induces brain functional connectivity changes in relapsing remitting multiple sclerosis patients: An exploratory study. Journal of Neurology. 2015;**262**:91-100

[60] Cerasa A, Gioia MC, Valentino P, et al. Computer assisted cognitive rehabilitation of attention deficits for multiple sclerosis: A randomized trial with fMRI correlates. Neurorehabilitation and Neural Repair. 2013;**27**:284-295

[61] Mattioli F, Stampatori C, Bellomi F, et al. A RCT comparing specific intensive cognitive training to aspecific psychological intervention in RRMS: The SMICT study. Frontiers in Neurology. 2015;**5**:278

[62] Mattioli F, Bellomi F, Stampatori C, et al. Two years follow up of domain specific cognitive training in relapsing remitting multiple sclerosis: A randomized clinical trial. Frontiers in Behavioral Neuroscience. 2016;**10**:28

[63] Das Nair R, Martin K, Lincoln NB. Memory rehabilitation for people with multiple sclerosis. Cochrane Database of Systematic Reviews. 2016;**3**:CD008754. DOI: 10.1002/14651858.CD008754.pub3

[64] Rosti-Otajarvi EM, Hamalainen PI. Neuropsychological rehabilitation for multiple sclerosis. The Cochrane Database of Systematic Reviews. 2014; **11**:CD009131

Chapter 5

Language Disorders in Multiple Sclerosis

Majid Soltani and Parvane Rahimifar

Abstract

Communicating ability is one of the necessary social needs in human, and language is a critical part of daily connections and communications. Language is impaired by different central nervous system (CNS) diseases such as multiple sclerosis (MS). MS leads to a language disorder by creating some plaques in subcortical constructions such as naming problems, semantic errors, and circumlocutory naming errors, semantic paraphasia, nonfluent speech, and grammatical and syntactic problems such as reduced mean maximum length of sentences and the number of spoken words and impairment in high-level language skills.

Keywords: multiple sclerosis, language, language disorder

1. Introduction

Communicating ability is one of the necessary social needs in human, and language is a critical part of daily connections and communications. Hence, any disorders in language result in inappropriate transferring of thoughts, idea, needing others, and finally inappropriate communication. According to studies, language is disrupted in different ways through the central nervous system (CNS), including Parkinson's, Alzheimer's, amyotrophic lateral sclerosis (ALS), and multiple sclerosis [1–6]. MS leads to language disorder by creating some plaques in language-related areas. If not treated, these disorders limit social life, professional life, mental life, and quality of life [7, 8]. If language disorders not treated, these disorders limit social, professional, mental, and quality of life. It is necessary to get involved with language interventions at the early stages of the disease and immediately after the detection of language disorders if life quality of MS patients is to be protected. Early detection and intervention in language disorders in these patients result in fast improvements in language functions, preventing the development of these disorders and finally preserving daily communication, social, functional, and professional life quality. Language interventions at the early stages of MS disease require accurate awareness of every kind of language disorders and the detection of various language disorders. Therefore, given the importance of language in daily communications, and social, professional, and functional lives, it is necessary to know language and its composing subsystems and various language disorders in MS disease. Note that detecting these disorders helps language and speech pathologists, neurologists, and other rehabilitation and MS-related specialists to be useful in early intervention and prevention of quality of life decreasing in MS patients. Therefore, in this chapter, we discuss language disorders in MS, language disorder detection history, and various language disorders in these patients.

2. What is language?

Language is a social code or a conventional system to reflect concepts through using conventional symbols and the rules related to combining these symbols [9]. As shown in **Figure 1**, language is complex, and a multiple-level phenomenon consisted of three main aspects; form, content, and use [10]. In other words, language is a complex cognitive function including pragmatic, semantic, syntax, morphology, and phonology subsystems (more information in **Table 1**).

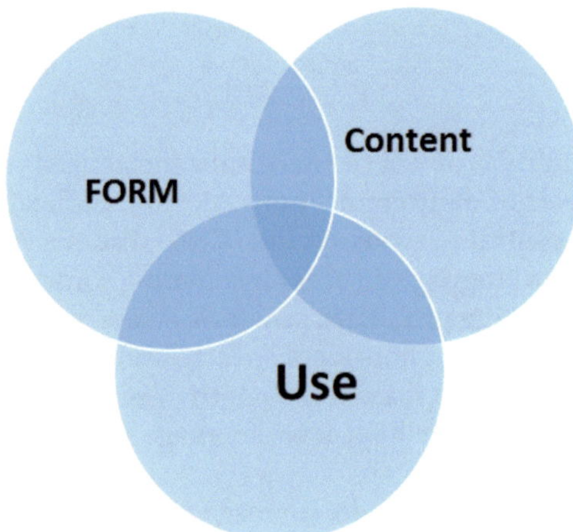

Figure 1.
The three main aspects.

Linguistic system	Deficits
Phonology Phonology is the study of the sound system of language, and includes the rules that govern its spoken form. Phonology analyzes which sound units are within a language and examines how these sounds are arranged, their systematic organization and rule system.[17]	• Frequently appear as articulation disorders. • Subject omits a consonant: "oo" for you • Subject substitutes one consonant: "wabbit" for rabbit • Discrimination: subject hears "go get the nail" instead of mail
Morphology Morphology is the study of the structure of words; it analyzes how words are built out of morphemes, the basic unit of morphology. Morpheme is the smallest meaningful unit of a language.[17]	• Subject may not use appropriate inflectional endings in their speech (e.g.,"He walk" or "Mommy coat"). • Subject may lack irregular past tense or irregular plurals (e.g., "drived" for "drove" or "mans" for "men"). Be aware of "Black English": "John cousin" "fifty cent", or "She work here".
Syntax Syntax consists of organizational rules denoting word, phrase, and clause order. It also examines the organization and relationship between words, word classes, grammar of the language and other sentence elements.[17]	• Lack the length or syntactic complexity (e.g., "Where Daddy go?"). • Problems comprehending sentences that express relationship between direct or indirect objects. Difficulty with wh questions. Difficulty with grammar of language (e.g. " mum went to work everyday)
Semantics Semantics is the study of linguistic meaning and includes the meaning of words, phrases, and sentences.[17]	• Limited vocabulary especially in adjectives, adverbs, prepositions, or pronouns. • Longer response time in selecting vocabulary words. • Fail to perceive subtle changes in word meaning: incomplete understanding and misinterpretations. • Figurative language problems.
Pragmatics Pragmatic is the study of knowledge and ability to use language functionally in social or interactive situations and integrates all the other language skills, but also requires knowledge and use of rule governing the use of language in social context.	• Problems understanding indirect requests (e.g., may say yes when asked "Must you play the piano?"). • May enter conversations in a socially unacceptable fashion or fail to take turns talking. • Difficulty staying on topic.

Ref. [55].

Table 1. *Description of language measures. Ref. [55].*

3. What is language disorder?

The American Speech-Language-Auditory Association (ASHA) considers any disorder in comprehension and applying symbolic speech, writing, and another symbolic system as a language disorder. This may occur in any of the three main language aspects (form, content, use) in semantic, syntax, morphology, phonology, and pragmatic subsystems (**Table 1**).

4. Language disorders in MS disease

Multiple sclerosis (MS) is a type of progressive central nervous system disease in which myelin sheaths are destroyed, and plaques are created in some parts of the brain and spinal cord's white material [11]. MS is the most common neurologic disease in people aging 20–45, and its prevalence is four times more in women than in men. Depending on the country and its special population, its prevalence is 2–150 individuals per 100,000 individuals [12]. According to the Multiple Sclerosis International Federation report in 2015, 2,300,000 million people in the world suffer from the MS disease [3]. Common symptoms of the disease include physical and sensory movement problems, speech disorders such as dysarthria, cognitive disorders, and language disorders [11].

5. Language disorder history in MS

In the recent two decades, researchers believed that MS harms subcortical areas, and cortical disorder causes language deficits [7, 13]. For this, no research was done on MS cognitive functions in the language field. However, along with brain imaging developments, it is proved that not only are subcortical structures such as the thalamus, caudate nucleus, globus pallidus, subthalamic nucleus, substantia nigra, and cerebellum effective in adjusting and coordinating the movement aspects of speech, but also they play a role in the processing of cognitive and language functions [14]. Using PET scan, some researchers showed that the thalamus and basal ganglia start to work during doing language assignments like picture naming [15] and word repeating [14, 16]. Using FMRI, Crosson et al. found a remarkable activity in subcortical structures while doing some language skills [14, 17]. Therefore, considering the researches, we can conclude that not only brain cortical but also subcortical structures, including the thalamus and its other structures and cerebellum, play a role in language processing and cause language disorders in MS patients [14, 18]. Another issue showing the possibility of language deficits in MS patients is cognitive deficits, as cognitive skills (memory and attention) are related to language skills [19, 20]. Memory disorder is one of the MS's common symptoms causing problems in information retrieving and decoding [20, 21]. In addition, memory disorder affects language assignments including verbal fluency [22], naming [23], and language comprehension [21, 24].

6. Language disorder types in MS

Studies show that individuals with progressive neurologic diseases such as MS experience not only have speech production deficits but also language problems [7]. Although some researchers confirm various language disorders in MS, they believe that these disorders are prevalent [3].

Language disorder means any disorder to the semantic, syntax, morphology, phonology, and pragmatic abilities appearing in different forms with different severities.

Among the existing language disorders, naming problems [1, 23, 25–27], verbal fluency [1, 8, 23, 28] in language production, and syntax skills including maximum sentence length mean reduction, word number reduction [18, 29], and deficiency in high-level language skills [7, 18, 30] are disorders seen in MS patients. Thus, regarding the special definition of each language disorder, we discuss each language disorder in MS separately.

7. Naming problem and verbal fluency deficit

The naming process is one of the basic lingual processes related to speech content and concept transfer. Naming is the person's ability to comprehend a visual symbol and retrieve its name correctly [31].

Naming deficit is one of the language disorders resulted from deficit in message content production [32] causing individual disability in achieving phonology and semantic characteristics from mental lexical storage [33]. Naming ability disorder is caused by different diseases [34], one of which is MS [1, 23, 25–27, 35]. In structural and functional changes in the brain and language path disorder, MS results in naming deficit [21], semantic error, circumlocution [36], and semantic paraphasia [24]. There are different reasons for justifying the naming ability deficit. Some researchers found insufficient memory [23], depression, and medicine intake. However, a particular relationship between medicine and language disorder is not confirmed yet [21]. Murdoch et al. found that the naming deficit is related to semantic disorders [21]. Le Dorze et al. pointed that retrieving semantic information deficit is related to cognitive problems like attention and memory in these patients [37]. However the relationship between cognitive and naming disorders is a challenge [21].

The naming disorder's severity can be different depending on the disease progress; sometimes a more severe disease may cause a more severe naming disorder and directly affect individual's daily functions [21].

There are various tasks to evaluate naming disorders, including confrontational naming, naming semantic levels, automatic serial naming, repetition, and verbal fluency [38].

Verbal fluency is a cognitive function facilitating information retrieval from the memory. It is also sensitive to cognitive disorders caused by the brain's dysfunction [39], involving the evaluation of the related processes in the naming process, including accessing lexical and semantic information [40]. Verbal fluency is disrupted after various diseases such as MS [1, 8, 23, 28]. MS results in verbal fluency disorder through caudate nuclei atrophy [39, 41], thalamus disorder, and basal ganglia [7, 42]. Henry and Beatty consider verbal fluency disorder as a common language disorder in MS patients [43].

8. Language production and syntax skill deficit

As mentioned earlier, language consisted of three main aspects: form, content, and use. Form includes grammar. Grammar refers to the knowledge of examining a language structure. Grammar has two components: morphology and syntax. Morphology studies words and phrase construction and is related to words' inner structures. Syntax is related to the order of elements in speech.

The evaluation proposed for the syntax structure of sentences in neurologic patients provides important information about neural instantiation and the organization of language [44]. Any disorder in grammar affects an individual's ability in transferring concepts in an exact sentence form [45].

There are various methods to study morpho-syntax skills, such as studying continuous speech and the elicitation procedure.

In most studies, continuous speech and sentence completion analysis methods are used to examine morpho-syntax skills so far. The continuous speech method can be administered in two ways: soliloquy and conversation. Researchers believe that soliloquy is better, as speech-language pathologists speak less and soliloquy writing is easier [18]. Being able to define language problems through this method, soliloquy needs a high degree of linguistic-cognitive interactions [29, 46].

Some clinical measures for syntactic complexity are used to analyze continuous speech in these studies, including the mean length of utterance in morphemes (MLU), mean clauses per utterance (MCU), developmental sentence scoring (DSS), remediation and screening procedure analysis (LARSP), the syntactic complexity score (SCS), and the picture-elicited scoring procedure for LARSP (PSL). MLU is one of the informal measures in continuous speech analysis applied in several studies to examine adults' syntax complexity [47–50]. Some scholars reported a meaningful difference between patients and healthy people's syntax skills. These measures are also used to study syntax skills in MS patients compared to healthy people [18, 29]. Some mentioned no deficit in syntax skills [51, 52]. In the following, we will discuss this in more details.

MCU is a useful measure and shows the number of conjoined and embedded clauses in a speech used to study syntax complexity in speaking in adults [48–51].

DSS is a valuable tool to evaluate grammar growth, help diagnostic judgments, help plan treatment, and evaluate treatment results [53]. This measure is used to examine syntax complexity skills in adults in various studies [48–50]. Another group of researchers applied this measure to study syntax skills in MS patients [51, 52]. This is mentioned in MLU findings.

Being useful for kids and adults, LARSP is a method to describe syntax complexity in a language sample, ability on the clauses, subordinate clause, phrase and word levels, and grammatical abilities [54]. Two scales, SCS and PSL, are used in this method. SCS calculates the number of grammatical categories (subject, verb, object, and complement) in a speech. Single-word speech does not include syntax skills, and syntax is composed of the relationship between morphemes. SCS is only used to calculate multiword utterances [51]. PSL is another measure of syntax complexity applied to facilitate the scoring of the Renfrew Action Picture Test (RAPT) [51]. Only one study used the LARSP profile and SCS and PSL to examine syntax skills in MS patients and showed no deficit in these patients [51].

The investigations showed that grammar deficit is one of the language disorders in MS patients [18, 29, 55, 56]. In defining syntax deficits, they also showed that MS patients demonstrate a combination of syntax-semantic disorders [55]. Morphology is one of the language components playing an important role in syntax phrase, since there is a relationship between morphology and syntactic components and they can appear as syntax [55]. To show this, various studies demonstrated that MS patients have syntactic errors resulted from morphologic errors [29, 55]. Studies on grammar in MS patients each showed a type of deficit in syntax skills. One of these deficits was shorter sentences, decrease in the word number mean, and the most spoken words in a sentence. Researchers pointed that MS patients have language structure deficits related to cognitive impairment, especially administrative function impairment. However, the role of aphasia on such disorders cannot be denied [18]. In another study, researchers showed that the number of sentences mean and the length of the longest sentence decrease. However, there was not a meaningful difference in sentence length mean between MS patients and healthy people. This is because of mild severity of the disease and no cognitive impairment [57] .

The elicitation procedure is another method to investigate morpho-syntax skill, one of which is sentence repetition skill being a fast method to provide information from an individual speech. The individual is asked to repeat whatever the pathologist says [58]. Although this method is criticized, evidence shows that with a high compatibility in their sentence repetition function with their self-motivated grammar level, if kids or adults have brain impairment, they will have better progress in the treatment. In cases where there is time limitation in evaluation and detection of patients' abilities, sentence repetition is a useful strategy for pathologist to gain information about individual ability in a short time [58].

Another advantage of sentence repetition is that it is easily implemented. Moreover, control, implementation, and analysis are more allowed in this method [59]. This method allows concentration on special grammar and phonology aspects, and they can be studied accurately. Researchers believe that sentence repetition assignment is a method with a high validity and reliability to evaluate general grammar knowledge (morphology, syntax) [59], and it is a valid language-psychology representation to detect language impairments [60]. So, we should use easy-implemented methods and immediately detect speech and language disorders to evaluate grammar structure. Based on this, among studies on syntax skill investigation, a study was implemented on MS patients using the long sentences repetition test (the first subtest of the Persian test of investigating high-level language skills). The results showed that, compared to a healthy person, the number of spoken words by an MS patient decreases meaningfully, and a meaningful decrease in the number of functional words (proposition, conjunction, and plural sign) and of content words (noun and verb) is a syntax deficit in MS patients. Compared to healthy people, they omit these words more often [61].

However, some researchers concluded that MS patients are not different with the ordinary people in using syntax structures [51, 52]. It is because of MS mild severity or being in recover period. Meanwhile, if a deficit is seen in complex language structures in MS, it is approvable through natural language measurement tools [51].

9. High-level language skills

High-level language skills mean language production in sentence or discourse level compared to single-word level [62]. These skills include several assignments, ambiguous sentences, sarcastic comprehension and explanation, proverb, conclusion, sentence making, long sentence repetition, celebrity naming, word definition, complex grammatical sentence comprehension, and comprehension and explanation of differences and similarities, and they use many language fields and cognitive processes [30].

Another aspect affected by neurologic diseases is high-level language skills. These skills are created following the amount of myelin decrease and subcortical paths impairment. In addition, a possible reason of high-level language skill deficit in MS is disconnection of cortical and subcortical areas [30]. The primary symptoms of high-level language skills in MS patients are comprehension and explanation deficits. They are along with deficit symptoms in ambiguous sentences comprehension, sarcastic comprehension and explanation, proverb, conclusion, sentence making, long sentence repetition, celebrity naming, word definition, complex grammatical sentence comprehension, and comprehension and explanation of differences and similarities [7, 63]. Deficit in these skills may be predictive of brain impairments and certain degenerative dementias [64, 65].

There are a few studies on MS that influence on high-level language skills so far. Primary studies evaluate high-level language skills based on standard aphasia tests. Although these tests investigate language skills, they are not complex and sensitive enough to exactly define language disorders and high-level language skills in MS patients [27, 66]. Thus, high-level language skills were studied using the test of language competence (TLC) and the word test (TWT). The results showed that, compared to healthy people, MS patients had lower scores in these skills, and there are more severe language problems in chronic progressive MS patients than in recrudescent-recovering one [30]. It is worth noting that TCL and TWT only study four high-level language skills, including the comprehension of ambiguous sentences, conclusion, proverb, and sentence making, and are useful for the ages of 9–11/18 [7, 30, 66]. A test named BESS was used in another study in Sweden showing impairment in high-level language skills. This is the only Swedish test investigating all high-level language skills and is complex and sensitive enough to evaluate all high-level language skills in MS patients with no age limitation [7]. Laakso et al. investigated high language functions in Swedish MS patients. They found that MS patients have language difficulties in repetition of long sentences, inference, metaphor, logico-grammatical sentence comprehension, comprehension of ambiguous sentences, and word definition. BESS validity was investigated in the Persian language in 2017. Rahimifar et al. studied its Persian version's validity and reliability. After confirming this test as a valid and matched tool with racial, linguistic, cultural, social, and geographical features in Persian people, they study high-level language skills in Persian MS patients and found out that, like other languages, high-level language skills were impaired in MS patients [56]. These studies show that we can use BESS test for clinical goals and we can detect language deficits sooner. As a result, language deficits of patients with progressive diseases will be treated faster [7, 56].

10. Conclusion

The study conducted on MS patients shows that the linguistic skills of these patients are damaged. Language disorders in MS include naming, verbal fluency disorder, syntax skills, and lack of high-level language skills. Researchers have focused more on the naming and verbal fluency, which are related to semantic component of language, and other areas of the language, including the form and language use, have been neglected. Therefore, it is imperative that all language skills, including high-level language skills, be addressed in MS patients.

Author details

Majid Soltani* and Parvane Rahimifar
Speech Therapy Department, Ahvaz Jundishapur University of Medical Sciences, Ahvaz, Iran

*Address all correspondence to: majidsoltanist@gmail.com

References

[1] Drake M, Allegri R, Carra A. Language abnormalities in patients with multiple sclerosis. Neurologia (Barcelona, Spain). 2002;**17**(1):12-16

[2] Berg E, Björnram C, Hartelius L, Laakso K, Johnels B. High-level language difficulties in Parkinson's disease. Clinical Linguistics & Phonetics. 2003;**17**(1):63-80

[3] Renauld S, Mohamed-Saïd L, Macoir J. Language disorders in multiple sclerosis: A systematic review. Multiple Sclerosis and Related Disorders. 2016;**10**:103-111

[4] Grossman M, D'Esposito M, Hughes E, Onishi K, Biassou N, White-Devine T, et al. Language comprehension profiles in Alzheimer's disease, multi-infarct dementia, and frontotemporal degeneration. Neurology. 1996;**47**(1):183-189

[5] Ferris SH, Farlow M. Language impairment in Alzheimer's disease and benefits of acetylcholinesterase inhibitors. Clinical Interventions in Aging. 2013;**8**:1007

[6] Strong MJ, Grace GM, Orange J, Leeper HA. Cognition, language, and speech in amyotrophic lateral sclerosis: A review. Journal of Clinical and Experimental Neuropsychology. 1996;**18**(2):291-303

[7] Laakso K, Brunnegård K, Hartelius L, Ahlsén E. Assessing high-level language in individuals with multiple sclerosis: A pilot study. Clinical Linguistics & Phonetics. 2000;**14**(5):329-349

[8] Ebrahimipour M, Shahbeigi S, Jenabi M, Amiri Y, Kamali M. Verbal fluency performance in patients with multiple sclerosis. Iranian Journal of Neurology. 2008;**7**(21):138-142

[9] Owens RE Jr. Language Development: An Introduction. Pearson; 2015

[10] Paul R. Language Disorders from Infancy through Adolescence: Assessment & Intervention. Elsevier Health Sciences; 2007

[11] Chiaravalloti ND, DeLuca J. Cognitive impairment in multiple sclerosis. The Lancet Neurology. 2008;**7**(12):1139-1151

[12] Ebrahimipour M, Hatefi Ardakani H. Speech Therapy in MS. Tehran: Setayesh Hasti; 2010

[13] Summers M, Fisniku L, Anderson V, Miller D, Cipolotti L, Ron M. Cognitive impairment in relapsing-remitting multiple sclerosis can be predicted by imaging performed several years earlier. Multiple Sclerosis. 2007

[14] Murdoch BE, Whelan BM. Speech and Language Disorders Associated with Subcortical Pathology. Hoboken, NJ: Wiley; 2009

[15] Price C, Moore C, Humphreys G, Frackowiak R, Friston KJ. The neural regions sustaining object recognition and naming. Proceedings of the Royal Society of London B. 1996;**263**(1376):1501-1507

[16] Price CJ, Price C, Wise R, Warburton E, Moore C, Howard D, et al. Hearing and saying: The functional neuro-anatomy of auditory word processing. Brain. 1996;**119**(3):919-931

[17] Crosson B, Benefield H, Cato MA, Sadek JR, Moore AB, Wierenga CE, et al. Left and right basal ganglia and frontal activity during language generation: Contributions to lexical, semantic, and phonological processes. Journal of the International

Neuropsychological Society. 2003;**9**(7):1061-1077

[18] Arrondo G, Sepulcre J, Duque B, Toledo J, Villoslada P. Narrative speech is impaired in multiple sclerosis. European Neurological Journal. 2010;**2**(1):11-40

[19] Denney DR, Gallagher KS, Lynch SG. Deficits in processing speed in patients with multiple sclerosis: Evidence from explicit and covert measures. Archives of Clinical Neuropsychology. 2011;**26**(2):110-119

[20] De Sonneville L, Boringa J, Reuling I, Lazeron R, Ader H, Polman C. Information processing characteristics in subtypes of multiple sclerosis. Neuropsychologia. 2002;**40**(11):1751-1765

[21] Pérez BdD. Anomia in People with Relapsing-Remitting Multiple Sclerosis. 2016

[22] Langdon DW. Cognition in multiple sclerosis. Current Opinion in Neurology. 2011;**24**(3):244-249

[23] Friend KB, Rabin BM, Groninger L, Deluty RH, Bever C, Grattan L. Language functions in patients with multiple sclerosis. The Clinical Neuropsychologist. 1999;**13**(1):78-94

[24] Klugman TM, Ross E. Perceptions of the impact of speech, language, swallowing, and hearing difficulties on quality of life of a group of south African persons with multiple sclerosis. Folia Phoniatrica et Logopaedica. 2002;**54**(4):201-221

[25] Beatty WW, Monson N. Lexical processing in Parkinson's disease and multiple sclerosis. Journal of Geriatric Psychiatry and Neurology. 1989;**2**(3):145-152

[26] Kujala P, Portin R, Ruutiainen J. Language functions in incipient cognitive decline in multiple sclerosis. Journal of the Neurological Sciences. 1996;**141**(1):79-86

[27] Lethlean JB, Murdoch BE. Naming errors in multiple sclerosis: Support for a combined semantic/perceptual deficit. Journal of Neurolinguistics. 1994;**8**(3):207-223

[28] Feinstein A. The Clinical Neuropsychiatry of Multiple Sclerosis. Cambridge: Cambridge University Press; 2007

[29] Jamalpour S, Baharlooie N, Ashtari F, Shamsian F, Sedehi M. Comparison some of the syntactic skills in Relapsing Remitting Multiple sclerosis and normal adults resident in Esfahan Province. Journal of Research Rehabilitation Sciences. 2013;**9**(5):866-875. [persian]

[30] Lethlean JB, Murdoch BE. Performance of subjects with multiple sclerosis on tests of high-level language. Aphasiology. 1997;**11**(1):39-57

[31] Wolf M, Denckla MB. RAN/RAS: Rapid Automatized Naming and Rapid Alternating Stimulus Tests. Austin, TX: Pro-ed; 2005

[32] Hallowell B, Chapey R, Chapey R. Language Intervention Strategies in Aphasia and Related Neurogenic Communication Disorders. Philadelphia: Lippincott, Williams, & Wilkins; 2008

[33] Bormann T, Blanken G, Wallesch C-W. 10 Mechanisms of lexical selection and the anomias. In: Ball M, Damico J, editors. Clinical Aphasiology: Future Directions: A Festschrift for Chris Code. Hove and New York: Psychology Press-Taylor and Francis Group; 2007. p. 156

[34] Raymer AM, Rothi L, Hillis A. Clinical diagnosis and treatment of naming disorders. The Handbook of Adult Language Disorders. 2002. pp. 163-182

[35] Tallberg I, Bergendal G. Strategies of lexical substitution and retrieval in multiple sclerosis. Aphasiology. 2009;**23**(9):1184-1195

[36] McDonald W, Ron M. Multiple sclerosis: The disease and its manifestations. Philosophical Transactions of the Royal Society of London Series B: Biological Sciences. 1999;**354**(1390):1615-1622

[37] Le Dorze G, Nespoulous J-L. Anomia in moderate aphasia: Problems in accessing the lexical representation. Brain and Language. 1989;**37**(3):381-400

[38] Chapey R. Language Intervention Strategies in Adult Aphasia. Baltimore, MD: Williams & Wilkins; 1986

[39] Kosmidis MH, Bozikas VP, Vlahou CH, Kiosseoglou G, Giaglis G, Karavatos A. Verbal fluency in institutionalized patients with schizophrenia: Age-related performance decline. Psychiatry Research. 2005;**134**(3):233-240

[40] Troyer AK. Normative data for clustering and switching on verbal fluency tasks. Journal of Clinical and Experimental Neuropsychology. 2000;**22**(3):370-378

[41] DeLuca GC, Yates RL, Beale H, Morrow SA. Cognitive impairment in multiple sclerosis: Clinical, radiologic and pathologic insights. Brain Pathology. 2015;**25**(1):79-98

[42] Mesulam M-M. Primary progressive aphasia—A language-based dementia. New England Journal of Medicine. 2003;**349**(16):1535-1542

[43] Henry JD, Beatty WW. Verbal fluency deficits in multiple sclerosis. Neuropsychologia. 2006;**44**(7):1166-1174

[44] Thompson CK, Fix S, Gitelman D. Selective impairment of morphosyntactic production in a neurological patient. Journal of Neurolinguistics. 2002;**15**(3-5):189-207

[45] Mehri A, Tahan Zadeh B, Jahani Y. Use of tense in Persian agrammatic Broca's aphasia. Bimonthly Audiology-Tehran University of Medical Sciences. 2010;**19**(1):78-85

[46] Arnott W, Jordan F, Murdoch B, Lethlean J. Narrative discourse in multiple sclerosis: An investigation of conceptual structure. Aphasiology. 1997;**11**(10):969-991

[47] Cheung H, Kemper S. Competing complexity metrics and adults' production of complex sentences. Applied Psycholinguistics. 1992;**13**(1):53-76

[48] Kemper S, Herman R, Lian C. Age differences in sentence production. The Journals of Gerontology Series B: Psychological Sciences and Social Sciences. 2003;**58**(5):P260-P8

[49] Kemper S, Herman RE, Liu C-J. Sentence production by young and older adults in controlled contexts. The Journals of Gerontology: Series B. 2004;**59**(5):220-224

[50] Kemper S, Thompson M, Marquis J. Longitudinal change in language production: Effects of aging and dementia on grammatical complexity and propositional content. Psychology and Aging. 2001;**16**(4):600

[51] Alma King K. Syntactic Complexity in Persons with and without Multiple Sclerosis. A Thesis Submitted for the Degree of Master of Science. Department of Communication Disorders. Brigham Young University; 2010

[52] Bjorkman KD. Variability of Syntactic Complexity in Persons With and Without Multiple Sclerosis. 2010

[53] Hughes DL, Fey ME, Long SH. Developmental sentence scoring: Still

useful after all these years. Topics in Language Disorders. 1992

[54] Crystal D. Working with LARSP. 1979

[55] Sonkaya AR, Bayazit ZZ. Language aspects of patients with multiple sclerosis. Eurasian Journal of Medicine and Investigation. 2018;**2**(3):133-138

[56] Rahimifar P, Soltani M, Madjdi Nasab N, Latifi M. Equivalent intercultural and evaluate the psychometric properties of the Persian version of the high-level language test (BESS) [thesis]. Ahvaz, Iran: Submitted for the degree of Master of Science, Dep of Speech Therapy Ahvaz Jundishapur University Of Medical Sciences; 2016

[57] Tomblin JB, Morris HL, Spriestersbach D. Diagnosis in Speech-Language Pathology. Singular Publishing Group; 1994

[58] Crain S, Thornton R. Investigations in Universal Grammar: A Guide to Experiments on the Acquisition of Syntax and Semantics. MIT Press; 2000

[59] Conti-Ramsden G, Botting N, Faragher B. Psycholinguistic markers for specific language impairment (SLI). Journal of Child Psychology and Psychiatry. 2001;**42**(6):741-748

[60] Batse E, Bretherton I, Snyder L. From First Word to Grammar: Individual Differences and Dissociable Mechanism. Cambridge: Cambridge University Press; 1988

[61] Rahimifar P, Soltani M, Moradi N, Majdi Nasab N, Latifi M. A comparative study of repetition of long sentences skill in Persian-speaking multiple sclerosis patients and healthy subjects. Koomesh Journal. 2017;**19**(1):122-128

[62] Murdoch BE, Theodoros DG. Speech and Language Disorders in Multiple Sclerosis. London: Whurr; 2000

[63] Keenan J. The detection of minimal dysphasia. Archives of Physical Medicine and Rehabilitation. 1971;**52**(5):227

[64] Faber-Langendoen K, Morris JC, Knesevich JW, LaBarge E, Miller JP, Berg L. Aphasia in senile dementia of the Alzheimer type. Annals of Neurology. 1988;**23**(4):365-370

[65] Crosson B. Assessment of subtle language deficits in neuropsychological batteries: Strategies and implications. In: Ecological Validity of Neuropsychological Testing. Delray, FL: GR Press/St Lucie Press, Inc; 1996

[66] Sanderson CE. Book review: Test of language competence. Journal of Psychoeducational Assessment. 1992;**10**(2):190-195

Section 5

Therapeutical Approach

Chapter 6

Non-Pharmacologic Therapies

Seyyedeh Zahra Safi

Abstract

The aim of this chapter is to assess the effectiveness of non-pharmacologic therapies like progressive muscle relaxation therapy (PMRT) as an adjunctive therapy for reducing level of depression for multiple sclerosis (MS) patients. One of the most common mood disorders is major depressive disorder (MDD) that MS patients experience it during their lives. MDD can exacerbate the symptoms of the MS disease. Non-pharmacologic therapies were held for the MS patients, twelve sessions of PMRT using Bernstein and Borkovec's method in spring 2010. According to the results, PMRT is effective in reducing depression. This therapy enables patients to reach relaxation quickly and thus can cope with depression reactions effectively.

Keywords: non-pharmacologic therapies, multiple sclerosis, depression, progressive muscle relaxation therapy

1. Introduction

These days the goal of all current and emerging therapeutic strategies for multiple sclerosis (MS) patients is to return them to a normal life despite of the disease [1].

Currently there is not any definitive treatment for MS disease and medications only reduce relapse rate, prolong remission, limit the onset of new MS lesions, and postpone the development of long-term disability [2].

Pharmacologic therapies (modafinil, dalfampridine, baclofen, diazepam, gabapentin, opioids) are used for symptomatic treatment of disability and symptoms, but these do not improve disease outcome [2].

The cause and cure is unknown; appearing, removing and even relapsing of symptoms occurs without any signs warning [3] and the onset of the disease may be acute or gradual [1]. Strong evidence for irreversible neurological disability in MS patients indicates that MS disease is an autoimmune disease against central nervous system myelin or neuron degeneration [4].

MS disease may prevent from some patients activities such as; employment, relationships (social, familial), goals and long term plans and activities of daily living [3]. Therefore these disabilities will challenge persons with MS disease, when they are attempting to pursue an active and compatible lifestyle [5].

Variable courses in MS disease are common. Within two to three decades, this disease changes from recoverable to unrecoverable neurological disorder and stable disability [6].

One million people in the world suffer from MS disease that has been reported 1.8 times more in females than males. MS is co morbid with psychiatric disorders and has a profound effect on the personal lives of individuals [7, 8].

IntechOpen

The psychosocial factors are closely associated with MS onset and may play important roles in the development of the disease [9].

MS disease usually indicates disparate disease periods and interaction between medical and psychological variables in MS disease is complex [7].

People with multiple sclerosis (MS) often report depression, poor sleep, fatigue, sleepiness and cognitive dysfunction. Interrelationships between symptoms are poorly understood [10].

For example findings suggest that treatment for depression is associated with reductions in the severity of fatigue symptoms [11] and many patients with multiple sclerosis (MS) report that stress can exacerbate disease [12].

Cognitive impairment is common in this disease [13]. Prevalence of cognitive impairment is about 30.5% and affects attention, concentration, performance, processing speed and visual perception [14].

These data point out the importance of orienting therapeutic interventions. For managing the symptoms of MS disease and improving or maintaining function and preserving the patient's quality of life are recommended careful clinical monitoring and pharmacologic and non-pharmacologic therapies [15].

Non-pharmacologic therapeutic strategies include psychotherapy, cognitive behavioral therapy, strengthen of coping, progressive muscle relaxation therapy (PMRT), etc. [16].

Non-pharmacologic therapies are used widely by MS patients and progressive muscle relaxation therapy (PMRT) is a form of complementary therapies [17].

For the first time Jacobson in 1934 recognized that the mind and selected muscles (16 muscle groups) work together in a united way. It means body can be relaxed with mental relaxation and mind can be relaxed with progressive muscle relaxation therapy (PMRT) [18].

This procedure was suited by Wolpe (1948) for systematic desensitization therapy and by Bernstein and Borkovec for stress management in cognitive-behavioral therapy in 1973. The Bernstein and Borkovec forms are brief and adapted that these are used generally (7 or 4 muscles groups) [18, 19].

In fact, relaxation therapy is several methods to show patients how they can achieve relaxation. Most programs include training special breathing and progressive muscle relaxation (tension-release cycles) to reduce physical and mental tension [20].

The relaxation response is a physiological state and incompatible response against stress response [21] and has a significant psychological impact on specific aspects of our personality and changing unwanted habits and attitudes [22].

Muscle tension is associated with stress and anxiety, which are related with depression strongly [20]. Depression had a negative impact on all quality of life domains and anxiety impact on mental domains [23].

It seems that unpredictable courses of disease activity influence in many different fields of their life. Unpredictable periods can make severe feelings of helplessness and depression in patients with MS [7], also the hopelessness hypothesis states that unpredictable and negative events of life patients leads to depression [24].

Depression is the predominant psychological disturbance with lifetime prevalence around 50% and annual prevalence of 20%. With diagnosis of MS, anxiety increases and depression is commoner during relapses also increases the rate of suicidal ideation and treating depression improves adherence to disease-modifying drugs [25].

MS patients often hide symptoms of depression and they complain from other symptoms [26]. Therefore treatment plans for depression among MS patients should be treated with individual and integrated approach [25].

According to the American Psychological Association (2018), people with depression may experience a lack of interest and pleasure in daily activities, inability to concentrate, feelings of worthlessness or excessive guilt and recurrent thoughts of death or suicide (non-somatic symptoms), significant weight loss or gain, insomnia or excessive sleeping, lack of energy (somatic symptoms).

Significant results show that PMRT, helpfulness for human suffering from depression in groups with brain health (different patients, like: multiple somatoform syndrome, cancer disease, pulmonary disease, cardiac disease, muscular pain, tinnitus disease and night eating syndrome) and brain lesion (MS patients).

Treatment by PMRT for depression is better than no-treatment or placebo treatment or other behavioral methods treatment. The comparison between the first intervention and the follow up showed that the effect of the treatment remained (sometimes more) [27–39].

According to recent researches, it was assumed that PMRT may reduce the level of major depressive disorder in female MS patients in Shiraz Multiple Sclerosis Aid Society (SH.M.S.A.S).

2. Methods and materials

This study was an applied-experimental research with randomized controlled trial design plus pre and posttests.

Study included the independent variable (progressive muscle relaxation therapy PMRT) and dependent variable (depression).

This study compared two groups; experimental and control.

The first group received (PMRT) and the second group did not receive any treatment for depression.

In spring 2010, from 2800 MS patients in SH.M.S.A.S 30 female volunteers participated in this study.

They answered the questionnaire before the intervention (Beck Depression Inventory BDI-II).

Criteria of MS and major depressive disorder (MDD) disease from minimal to severe were confirmed by the SHMSAS and BDI-II.

After the pretest, cases were matched in terms such as: degree of depression age, marital status, education and income then randomly divided in two groups.

The experimental group received standard care for MS disease plus 60 min of psychological intervention (PMRT) for each session (twice a week for six weeks) by M.A Clinical Psychology in Society of MS.

The control group received only standard care for MS disease.

Until the end of the treatment, drop out did not occur in the number of patients and two groups cooperated again in the posttest (answered the questionnaire for the second time).

2.1 Rights and criteria

Ethical considerations and rights were applied for this research (respect to basic rights of patients such as; privacy, cultural and social values, freedom of choice and honesty about characteristics of therapy and therapist's competence).

Selection criteria:

1. Willing to attend in therapy meeting.

2. Having physical ability and minimal level of literacy was sufficient.

3. Accepting the philosophy of doing daily assignments and filling out weekly notes.

2.2 The content of therapy sessions

The best way for muscle relaxation is for muscles to be contracted as much as possible, and then be relaxed suddenly (tension-release sequence). The released force from the treatment increases the excitability threshold. The released force is a big step toward deeper relaxation and patients can understand the feeling of tension and relaxation of muscles (comparative judgment). Relaxation therapy was divided to two parts:

1. The first six sessions: special breathing plus contraction and relaxation of muscles, with gradual reduction of the number of muscles involved.

2. The second six sessions: special breathing plus contraction and relaxation of mind [21].

2.3 Tools

In this intervention for therapy meetings, Progressive Muscle Relaxation, was used by method of Bernstein and Borkovec, 1973 [18], also the Beck Depression Questionnaire (Beck, Epstein, Brown and Steer, 1988) was used, with the reliability (0.91) and validity (0.87) of the Iranian valid [40].

The BDI-II was expanded based on criteria of diagnostic and statistical manual of mental disorders, fourth edition (DSM-IV) for diagnosing depressive disorders [41].

The BDI-II is a brief scale that it is suitable for researchers as a screening tool. It is a subjective paper and pencil questionnaire with ordinal scale. In addition cut-off points (0–13), (14–19), (20–28) and (29–63) show minimal, mild, moderate and severe depression [41].

2.4 Iranian validation

Based on Iranian Validation, validity was certified by positive correlation, between Beck Depression Inventory (BDI-II) and Brief Symptom Inventory (BSI), coefficient of Pearson was 0.87, and factor analysis showed physical factor, cognitive factor and affective factor.

And reliability was certified by method of internal consistency, Cronbach's alpha coefficient was 0.91 [40].

2.5 Analysis method of data

To remove covariate variable was applied Analysis of Covariance and to remove difference between two groups was applied Levine Test.

In this intervention, the variables were Progressive Muscle Relaxation Therapy as independent and Depression as dependent variable after that analysis of Variance was applied with technique of Repeated Measures.

3. Results

Thirty MS patients attended in this intervention that they were separated randomly in two groups (experimental and control). **Tables 1** and **2** was designed for context variables and descriptive statistics of depression.

Table 1, shows half of patients in this intervention were sick more than 5 years and they had tolerated symptoms from mild to severe and they were in the third decade of their life and in status of marital single patients were more than others. Also in education degree most of them had a bachelor's degree.

All patients had depression and some of them had severe depression that in experimental group the mean value indicates mild depression (the results are raveled in **Table 2**).

The intervention hypothesis explains that PMRT may reduce the level of depressive disorder. This assumption was checked by **Tables 3–5**.

Table 3, was designed to measure the equality of variances between groups.

The results indicate that there was no significant difference in the variance of groups.

The purpose of Covariance Analysis in **Table 4** was to eliminate of the covariate variable from the dependent variable and to estimate the central indexes.

After intervention, with notice to the significance level and after omitting the impact of pretest on posttest, finding revealed the mean and standard deviation has increased (reduce depression). A significant reduction in depression variable occurred in seven levels.

In **Table 5**, Analysis of Variance with Repeated Measures method reviewed the impact of intervention on depression.

Table 5 showed that the difference between pretest and posttest was significant ($p = 0.0001$) and this difference was 49% reduction in depression levels, it means that this reduction has occurred because of the relaxation therapy and statistical power was 99%.

		Experimental group		Control group	
		Frequency	Percentage	Frequency	Percentage
Sick precedent	Less than 2 years	4	0.26	4	0.26
	2–5 years	2	0.13	3	0.20
	5–10 years	7	0.46	8	0.53
	More than 10 years	2	0.13	0	0.00
Age	Second decade	5	0.33	4	0.26
	Third decade	5	0.33	6	0.40
	Fourth decade	4	0.26	3	0.20
	Fifth decade	1	0.60	2	0.13
Marital status	Single	7	0.46	5	0.33
	Married	5	0.33	6	0.40
	Divorced	2	0.13	2	0.13
	Widow	1	0.60	2	0.13
Education degree	High school	3	0.20	4	0.26
	Diploma	4	0.26	5	0.33
	Bachelor	8	0.53	6	0.40
	Master	0	0.00	0	0.00

Table 1.
Context variable in experimental and control groups.

	Control		Experimental		Total	
	After	Before	After	Before	After	Before
Mean	15.93	15.86	8.40	16.20	12.16	16.03
Median	13	13	5	16	10	14
Mode	10	11	5	11	5	11
Sum	239	238	126	243	365	481
Std. deviation	9.72	9.76	9.43	9.50	10.16	9.46
Variance	94.49	95.26	88.9	90.31	103.24	89.62
Range	31	31	40	36	40	37
Maximum	34	34	40	40	40	40

Table 2.
Descriptive statistics of depression variable.

	F	First-degree of freedom	Second-degree of freedom	Significant level
Depression	0.463	1	28	0.502

Table 3.
Levine test results (about equal variances in the two groups).

Experimental group	Average	Standard deviation	Number	Average difference	Meaningful level
Before intervention	16.08	1.03	15	7.83	0.000
After intervention	8.24	1.03	15	−7.83	0.000

Table 4.
The estimate of average depression variable.

	Source of changes	Sig	Effect	Statistical power
Effects	Depression	0.0001	0.49	99
	Interaction depression and group	0.0001	0.55	99
	Error			

Table 5.
Results of variance analysis with repeated measures method.

4. Discussion

MS patients spent a lot of time to control emotional disorders, like depression. Levels of depression were studied by researchers and the results showed high levels of this variable and the effects of depression on MS disease exacerbation [42–59].

For example:

The possibility that the health status of negative mental can change period of MS disease since Charcot (1879, he was the first proposer), has been discussed, that shows grief and worry might influence on onset and exacerbation of disease symptoms [3].

Negative emotions (like depression) in the MS patients correlated with their family troubles and social isolation [9].

Non-somatic symptoms of depression can predict cognitive performance [14] and on the other hand somatic and non-somatic symptoms of depression predict exacerbation of MS disease [60].

Depression is an important predictor parameter on psychological balance of MS patients [61] and studies have confirmed that there are the relationships between structural brain lesions with depression in MS patients [24] and may be lesion site has two function: increases in depression and sleep disturbance (fatigue symptoms) [62].

Previous studies have indicated that depression is prevalent in MS patients and affects treatment adherence and associates with the neurologic damage that results from multiple sclerosis [42–59].

This study was designed to purpose that with identifying and treating the first symptoms of depression, patients can increase the performance of themselves in the society.

This study was designed to assess hypothesis derived from the Gate Theory this theory states that psychological factors influence on physical factors of pain [physical pain and psychological pain]. It means, the same way that stress and discomfort can exacerbate pain, relief and relaxation can also reduce pain [63] and depression is an overwhelming psychological pain [64], therefore this randomized controlled study during twelve sessions was carried out to determine the effects of treatment on experimental group. The results showed that there was a significant relationship between treatment and depression. **Table 4** shows mild depression in experimental group and after intervention average of depression reduction was seven levels; operationally it define that patients in experimental group indicated state of depression like normal people.

Analysis of Variance showed that these changes (it was 49%) in the group, were as a result of progressive muscle relaxation therapy.

Table 2 shows severe depression in some cases before and after treatment. They often hide symptoms of depression or cannot recognize between symptoms of depression and MS disease. Also previous treatments (like pharmacologic therapy) for severe depression were continued. These cases took less advantage from this treatment.

Measurement of depression in patients with MS is complicated because some of the symptoms are identical between depression and MS disease (excessive fatigue, cognitive difficulties, psychomotor retardation, mood changes, sleep changes and emotional changes) [65].

Findings of this study showed that the level of depression (first symptoms of depression), even in the short-term treatment has reduced, which were considered 6 weeks (as a safe, inexpensive and effective intervention) and demonstrated the effectiveness of PMRT in reducing depression as non-pharmacologic treatment, when treatment was used systematically.

Findings of this short-term treatment were consistent with the research of Jorm and Morgan [20]. They confirmed that PMRT as psychological intervention for depression patients are more acceptable than other interventions (relaxation imagery, autogenic training) and finding of Annette and Jens's study [66] demonstrated both cognitive behavioral therapy (CBT) and PMRT appear to be effective treatments for depression in the normal human brain.

Based on the results of Sutherland and Andersen [3] and Artemiadis and Vervainioti [39] and Molina and Pérez in Spain [67] and Ghafari and Ahmadi in Iran [68], potentially, it could be stated that PMRT may provide benefits in different dimensions of the disease (vitality, fatigue, depression) in the brain affected with MS.

However in psychological interventions, therapist training is essential. In fact, relaxation technique is an acceptable psychological intervention, which this method requires less skill and training than other techniques.

Finally, rationale and supporting evidence, and techniques used in Progressive Muscle Relaxation Therapy was summarized in this article for intuitive understanding of future researchers about influences of PMRT.

4.1 Suggestions

PMRT is effective treatment for depression in MS patients, although more studies should be done for investigating the relaxation therapy as a first-line treatment in a stepped care approach to managing depression in MS patients. Therefore, to obtain more accurate results, the following recommendations are given:

1. It is suggested that in future studies, should be used more objective clinical and laboratory studies.

2. More control of confounding variables can reduce the limitations of the study (such as: sex, social and cultural status and disease progression).

3. Quantity of therapy will be better by using tapes, movies or booklets and long-term treatment.

4. Finally, it is recommended screening programs for depression in MS disease for facilitating access to services for all MS patients.

Acknowledgements

All praise belongs to Allah (Alhamdulillah) for giving me an opportunity to complete this study. Allah bless and special greetings upon prophet, Mohammad (peace be upon him) and his household who has saved humanity from the darkness to the lightness.

This study dedicated to Hazrat Fateme-Zahra (peace be upon her), Emam Hosein (peace be upon him) chief of martyrs and Emam Mahdi (peace be upon him). Also this study dedicated to martyrs of the 8 years of the holy defense (martyr Seyyed Ahmad Safi, martyr Mohammad-Jafar Pourakbari, martyr Seyyed Mohammad Safi).

DOI: http://dx.doi.org/10.5772/intechopen.86288

Author details

Seyyedeh Zahra Safi[1,2]

1 Psychology and Counseling Organization of Islamic Republic of Iran, Shiraz, Islamic Republic of Iran

2 M.A Clinical Psychology, Member of Psychology and Counseling organization of Islamic Republic of Iran, Iran

*Address all correspondence to: safi5zohreh@gmail.com

References

[1] McCabe MP, McKern S. Quality of life and multiple sclerosis: Comparison between people with multiple sclerosis and people from the general population. Clinical Psychology in Medical Settings. 2002;**9**(4):287

[2] Tullman MJ. A review of current and emerging therapeutic strategies in multiple sclerosis. Managed Care. 2013;**19**(2):21-27

[3] Sutherland G, Andersen MB, Morris T. Relaxation and health-related quality of life in multiple sclerosis: The example of autogenic training. Behavioral Medicine. 2005;**28**(3):249-256

[4] Keegan BM, Noseworthy JH. Multiple sclerosis. Annual Review of Medicine. 2002;**53**:285-302

[5] White LJ, Dressendorfer RH. Exercise and multiple sclerosis. Sports Medicine. 2004;**34**(15):1077-1100

[6] Trapp BD, Nave KA. Multiple sclerosis: An immune or neurodegenerative disorder. Annual Review of Neuroscience. 2008;**31**:247-269

[7] Shnek ZM, Foley FW, LaRocca NG. Helplessness, self-efficacy, cognitive distortions and depression in multiple sclerosis and spinal cord injury. Annals of Behavioral Medicine. 1997;**19**(3):287-294

[8] Skokou M, Soubasi E, Gourzis P. Depression in multiple sclerosis: A review of assessment and treatment approaches in adult and pediatric populations. ISRN Neurology. 2012;**2012**:1-6

[9] Liu XJ, Ye HX, Li WP. Relationship between psychosocial factors and onset of multiple sclerosis. European Neurology. 2009;**62**(3):130-136

[10] Sater RA, Gudesblatt M, Kresa-Reahl K, Brandes DW, Sater PA. The relationship between objective parameters of sleep and measures of fatigue, depression, and cognition in multiple sclerosis. Multiple Sclerosis Journal Experimental, Translational and Clinical. 2015;**1**:1-8

[11] Mohr DC, Hart SL, Goldberg A. Effects of treatment for depression on fatigue in multiple sclerosis. Psychosomatic Medicine. 2003;**65**(4):542-547

[12] Mohr DC, Goodkin DE, Nelson S. Moderating effects of coping on the relationship between stress and the development of new brain lesions in multiple sclerosis. More Psychosomatic Medicine. 2002;**64**(5):803-809

[13] Hardmeier M, Schoonheim MM, Geurts JJ, Hillebrand A, Polman CH, Barkhof F, et al. Cognitive dysfunction in early multiple sclerosis: Altered centrality derived from resting-state functional connectivity using magneto-encephalography. PLoS ONE. 2012;**7**(7):420

[14] Sundgren M, Maurex L, Wahlin A, Piehl F, Brismar T. Cognitive impairment has a strong relation to non-somatic symptoms of depression in relapsing-remitting multiple sclerosis. Archives of Clinical Neuropsychology. 2013;**28**(2):144-155

[15] Crayton HJ, Rossman HS. Managing the symptoms of multiple sclerosis: A multimodal approach. Clinical Therapeutics. 2006;**28**(4):445-460

[16] JoséSá M. Psychological aspects of multiple sclerosis. Clinical Neurology and Neurosurgery. 2008;**110**(9):868-877

[17] Ghafari S, Ahmadi F, Nabavi M, Kazemnejad A, Memarian R, Rafatbakhsh M. Effectiveness of applying progressive muscle relaxation technique on quality of life of patients

with multiple sclerosis. Clinical Nursing. 2009;**18**(15):2171-2179

[18] Bernstein D, Borkovec T, Carlson K. In: Sahebi A, editor. Progressive Relaxation Training: A Manual for the Helping Professions. Mashhad: Ferdowsi University Press; 1992. Translated by Sahebi A (Persian)

[19] McCallie MS, Blum CM, Hood CJ. Progressive muscle relaxation. Human Behavior in the Social Environment. 2006;**13**(3):51-66

[20] Jorm AF, Morgan AJ, Hetrick SE. Relaxation for depression. Cochrane Database of Systematic Reviews. 2008;**8**(4):1-3

[21] Chang BH, Dusek JA, Benson H. Psychobiological changes from relaxation response elicitation: Long-term practitioners vs. novices. Psychosomatics. 2011;**52**(6):550-559

[22] Ramasamy S, Panneerselvam S, Govindharaj P, Kumar A, Nayak R. Progressive muscle relaxation technique on anxiety and depression among persons affected by leprosy. Exercise Rehabilitation. 2018;**14**(3):375-381

[23] Goretti B, Portaccio E, Zipoli V. Coping strategies, psychological variables and their relationship with quality of life in multiple sclerosis. Neurological Sciences. 2009;**30**(1):15-20

[24] Kneebone I, Dunmore E. Attributional style and symptoms of depression in persons with multiple sclerosis. Behavioral Medicine. 2004;**11**(2):110-115

[25] Schumann R, Adamaszek M, Sommer N, Kirkby KC. Stress, depression and antidepressant treatment options in patients suffering from multiple sclerosis. Current Pharmaceutical Design. 2012;**18**(36):5837-5845

[26] Alschuler KN, Ehde DM, Jensen MP. The co-occurrence of pain and depression in adults with multiple sclerosis. Rehabilitation Psychology. 2013;**58**(2):217-221

[27] Isa MR, Moy FM, Abdul Razack AH, Zainuddin ZM, Zainal NZ. Impact of applied progressive deep muscle relaxation training on the level of depression, anxiety and stress among prostate cancer patients: Quasi-experimental study. Asian Pacific Journal of Cancer Prevention. 2013;**14**(4):2237-2242

[28] Cafarella PA, effing TW, usmani Z-A, frith PA. Treatments for anxiety and depression in patients with chronic obstructive pulmonary disease: A literature review. Respirology. 2012;**17**(4):627-638

[29] Fernando LV, Angela T, Vanessa B, Olga D, Patricia O, Elisabet H. Comparison of relaxation training with a cognitive-behavioural intervention for indicated prevention of depression in university students: A randomized controlled trial. Psychiatric Research. 2012;**46**(11):1456-1463

[30] Hashim HA, Hanafi Ahmad Yusof H. The effects of progressive muscle relaxation and autogenic relaxation on young soccer players' mood states. Asian Journal of Sports Medicine. 2011;**2**(2):99-105

[31] Chang B, Casey A, Dusek JA, Benson H. Relaxation response and spirituality: Pathways to improve psychological outcomes in cardiac rehabilitation. Psychosomatic Research. 2010;**69**(2):93-100

[32] Lolak S, Connors GL, Sheridan MJ. Effects of progressive muscle relaxation training on anxiety and depression in patients enrolled in an outpatient pulmonary rehabilitation program. Psychotherapy and Psychosomatics. 2008;**77**(2):119-125

[33] Persson AL, Veenhuizen H, Zachrison L, Gard G. Relaxation as treatment for chronic muscular skeletal pain a systematic review of randomized controlled studies. Physical Therapy Reviews. 2008;**13**(5):355-365

[34] Pawlow LA, O'Neil PM, Malcolm RJ. Night eating syndrome: Effects of brief relaxation training on stress, mood, hunger, and eating patterns. Obesity. 2003;**27**(8):970-978

[35] McGrady AV, Kern-Buell C, Bush E, Devonshire R, Claggett AL, Grubb BP. Biofeedback-assisted relaxation therapy in neurocardiogenic syncope: A pilot study. Applied Psychophysiology and Biofeedback. 2003;**28**(3):183-192

[36] Sloman R. Relaxation and imagery for anxiety and depression control in community patients with advanced cancer. Cancer Nursing. 2002;**25**(6):432-435

[37] Weber C, Arck P, Mazurek B, Klapp BF. Impact of a relaxation training on psychometric and immunologic parameters in tinnitus sufferers. Psychosomatic Research. 2002;**52**(1):29-33

[38] Luebbert K, Dahme B, Hasenbring M. The effectiveness of relaxation training in reducing treatment-related symptoms and improving emotional adjustment in acute non-surgical cancer treatment: A meta-analytical review. Psycho-Oncology. 2001;**10**(6):490-502

[39] Artemiadis AK, Vervainioti AA, Alexopoulos EC, Rombos A, Anagnostouli MC, Darviri C. Stress management and multiple sclerosis: A randomized controlled trial. Archives of Clinical Neuropsychology. 2012;**27**(4):406-416

[40] Dabson KE, Mohamadkhani P. Psychometric characteristics of BDI-II in patients of MDD. Rehabilitation. 2007;**8**(29):104-111

[41] Wang YP, Gorenstein C. Assessment of depression in medical patients: A systematic review of the utility of the Beck depression inventory-II. Clinics (São Paulo, Brazil). 2013;**68**(9):1274-1287

[42] Firth N. Effectiveness of psychologically focused group interventions for multiple sclerosis: A review of the experimental literature. Health Psychology. 2014;**19**(6):789-801

[43] Stepleman LM, Decker M, Rollock M, Casillas R, Brands T. Depression screening in black Americans with multiple sclerosis. Psychology, Health & Medicine. 2014;**19**(1):33-39

[44] Tepavcevic DK, Pekmezovic T, Stojsavljevic N, Kostic J, Basuroski ID, Mesaros S, et al. Predictive value of health-related quality of life in progression of disability and depression in persons with multiple sclerosis: A 3-year study. Acta Neurologica Belgica. 2013;**113**(4):403-409

[45] Nielsen-Prohl J, Saliger J, Güldenberg V, Breier G, Karbe H. Stress stimulated volitional coping competencies and depression in multiple sclerosis. Psychosom Research. 2013;**74**(3):221-226

[46] Donnchadha OS, Burke T, Bramham J, O'Brien MC, Whelan R, Reilly R, et al. Symptom overlaps in anxiety and multiple sclerosis. Multiple Sclerosis. 2013;**19**(10):1349-1354

[47] Sarısoy G, Terzi M, Gümüş K, Pazvantoğlu O. Psychiatric symptoms in patients with multiple sclerosis. General Hospital Psychiatry. 2013;**35**(2):134-140

[48] Wood B, van der Mei IA, Ponsonby AL, Pittas F, Quinn S, Dwyer T, et al. Prevalence and concurrence of anxiety, depression and fatigue over time in multiple sclerosis. Multiple Sclerosis. 2013;**19**(2):217-224

[49] Jones KH, Ford DV, Jones PA, John A, Middleton RM, Lockhart-Jones H, et al. A large-scale study of anxiety and depression in people with multiple sclerosis: A survey via the web portal of the UK MS register. PLoS ONE. 2012;7(7):419

[50] Ghajarzadeh M, Sahraian MA, Fateh R, Daneshmand A. Fatigue, depression and sleep disturbances in Iranian patients with multiple sclerosis. Acta Medica Iranica. 2012;**50**(4):244-249

[51] Sjonnesen K, Berzins S, Fiest K.M, M Bulloch A.G, Metz L.M, Thombs B.D and Patten S.B. Evaluation of the 9-item patient health questionnaire (PHQ-9) as an assessment instrument for symptoms of depression in patients with multiple sclerosis. Postgraduate Medicine 2012;**124**(5):69-77

[52] Pozzilli C, Schweikert B, Ecari U, Oentrich W, Bugge JP. Quality of life and depression in multiple sclerosis patients: Longitudinal results of the BetaPlus study. Neurologija. 2012;**259**(11):2319-2328

[53] Dubayova T, Krokavcova M, Nagyova I, Rosenberger J, Gdovinova Z, Middel B, et al. Type D, anxiety and depression in association with quality of life in patients with Parkinson's disease and patients with multiple sclerosis. Quality of Life Research. 2013;**22**(6):1353-1360

[54] Fiest KM, Patten SB. The multiple sclerosis depression rating scale. Expert Review of Neurotherapeutics. 2012;**12**(9):1053-1055

[55] Labuz-Roszak B, Kubicka-Bączyk K, Pierzchała K, Machowska-Majchrzak A, Skrzypek M. Fatigue and its association with sleep disorders, depressive symptoms and anxiety in patients with multiple sclerosis. Neurologia i Neurochirurgia Polska. 2012;**46**(4):309-317

[56] Moore P, Hirst C, Harding KE, Clarkson H, Pickersgill TP, Robertson NP. Multiple sclerosis relapses and depression. Psychosom Research. 2012;**73**(4):272-276

[57] Brown RF, Valpiani EM, Tennant CC, Dunn SM, Sharrock M, Hodgkinson S, et al. Longitudinal assessment of anxiety, depression, and fatigue in people with multiple sclerosis. Psychology and Psychotherapy: Theory, Research and Practice. 2009;**82**(1):41-56

[58] Kehler MD, Hadjistavropoulos HD. Is health anxiety a significant problem for individuals with multiple sclerosis? Behavioral Medicine. 2009;**32**:150-161

[59] Tanaya NS, Rona M. Fatigue and social impairment in multiple sclerosis: The role of patients' cognitive and behavioral responses to their symptoms. Psychosomatic Research. 2006;**61**(5):587-593

[60] Burns MN, Nawacki E, Siddique J, Pelletier D, Mohr DC. Prospective examination of anxiety and depression before and during confirmed and pseudo exacerbations in patients with multiple sclerosis. Psychosomatic Medicine. 2013;**75**(1):76-82

[61] Chen K, Fan Y, Hu R, Yang T, Li K. Impact of depression, fatigue and disability on quality of life in Chinese patients with multiple sclerosis. Stress and Health. 2013;**29**(2):108-112

[62] Clark CM, Fleming JA. Sleep disturbance, depression, and lesion site in patients with multiple sclerosis. JAMA Neurology Arch Neurol. 1992;**49**(6):641-643

[63] Wilson P. Immediate Relief. Tehran: The Peykan Press; Translated by Tamadon T. 2000. Persian

[64] Sadok VA, Kaplan H. Kaplan and Sadock' Synopsis of Psychiatry: Behavioral Sciences–Clinical Psychiatry.

Tehran, Persian: The Shahre Abe Press; Translated by Poorafkari N. 2003

[65] Moran PJ, Mohr DC. The validity of Beck depression inventory and Hamilton rating scale for depression items in the assessment of depression among patients with multiple sclerosis. Behavioral Medicine. 2005;**28**(1):35

[66] Schröder A, Heider J, Zaby A. Cognitive behavioral therapy versus progressive muscle relaxation training for multiple somatoform symptoms: Results of a randomized controlled trial. Cognitive Therapy and Research. 2013;**37**:296-306

[67] Molina-Rueda F, Pérez de la Cruz S. Multiple sclerosis and relaxation techniques. Revista Iberoamericana Kinesiology and Physiotherapy. 2009;**12**(1):28-34. Spanish

[68] Ghafari S, Ahmadi F, Nabavi S.M, Memarian R and Kazemnejad A. Effect of applying progressive muscle relaxation on depression, anxiety and stress in multiple sclerosis patients. Iran Research in Medical Sciences. Persian. 2008;**32**(1):47-53

Chapter 7

Epstein-Barr Virus in Multiple Sclerosis

Gulfaraz Khan and Asma Hassani

Abstract

Multiple sclerosis (MS) is a chronic inflammatory disease of the central nervous system in which the body's immune system is abnormally directed towards the myelin sheaths covering the nerve fibers. What triggers the neuroinflammation and autoimmune destruction of the myelin sheaths remains unknown. However, it is widely accepted that susceptibility depends on a combination of genetic and environmental factors and their interactions. With little chance of influencing genetic predisposition, the importance of identifying risk factors which could be modulated to either prevent the on-set of MS or to ameliorate the course of the disease, is an attractive alternative. An accumulating body of evidence, including our own recent study involving over 1000 MS and non-MS samples, indicates that Epstein-Barr virus (EBV), a common herpesvirus, could be involved. In this chapter, we review the studies linking EBV to MS and propose an explanation by which this common virus could be involved in the pathogenesis of MS.

Keywords: multiple sclerosis, autoimmunity, neuroinflammation, Epstein-Barr virus, seroepidemiological evidence, postmortem studies

1. Introduction

Multiple sclerosis (MS) is a progressive disease in which multiple regions in the brain, spinal cord and optic nerve undergo myelin destruction or demyelination. It is believed that an aberrant immune response mistakenly attacks the myelin sheaths in the central nervous system (CNS) resulting in the formation of focal demyelinated plaques; the hallmark of MS [1]. In spite of extensive search, the identity of the factor(s) that triggers the immune assault against the myelin remains elusive. It is generally accepted that MS is a complex disease and most likely involves both genetic and environmental factors [2]. Although no single gene has been identified to be responsible in the development of MS, certain HLA haplotypes, such as HLA-DRB1 have been shown be associated with MS susceptibility [3]. Furthermore, the fact that MS is more prevalent in certain races such as Caucasians [4, 5] and incidence rates are increasing in some ethnic groups such as blacks [6, 7] supports the involvement of genes in the development of MS. Although the risk of MS is significantly higher in individuals with first-degree relatives with MS, this still does not explain the occurrence of MS in majority of cases. In fact, MS concordance in monozygotic twins is only around 25% [8, 9]. This clearly indicates that environmental factors play a key role in the development of MS in genetically predisposed individuals.

1.1 Environmental risk factors for MS

In support of the above observations, MS prevalence has been reported to be higher in the northern hemisphere, but lower towards the equator. However, recent studies indicate that this pattern of distribution, known as the latitudinal gradient, is changing in some countries such as Norway and USA [10–12]. Moreover, migration studies indicate that the increasing burden of MS is due to exposure to certain factors in the environment, which may account for a bigger proportion of MS risk than genetic factors. These studies show that leaving countries with high MS incidence prior to reaching adolescence, to regions with low MS incidence, confers protection against developing the disease [13]. Similarly, migrating in the opposite direction is linked to increased risk of developing MS [14–16]. These protective and MS predisposing effects have been shown to occur in a single generation, and this is highly unlikely to be due to effects of genes which usually manifest on longer periods of time [17].

Additionally, exposure to specific environmental agents at a young age seems to be critical in shaping the risk of developing MS [18]. The past few decades have seen a rapid accumulation of epidemiological data pointing to a number of different environmental factors that could potentially be involved in MS pathogenesis. However, no single causative agent has yet been unequivocally shown to be central to MS development [19]. Environmental risk factors associated with MS include sunlight exposure and serum levels of vitamin D, smoking, obesity, female sex hormones, and infection with Epstein-Barr virus (EBV) [20–22]. Among these factors, infection with EBV, particularly when manifested as infectious mononucleosis (IM), appears to have the most significant and consistent association with the risk of developing MS [23].

1.2 Infectious risk factors for MS: Hygiene hypothesis

The notion that an infectious agent is involved in the pathogenesis of MS is not new. A number of observations, including MS outbreak in the Faroes islands during World War II, which coincided with the British occupation of the islands [24], and MS occurrence in clustering fashion (e.g. familial clustering of MS), suggested an infectious cause for MS [17]. The hygiene hypothesis was used to provide an explanation for such involvement [21], assuming that certain infections occurring during the first few years of life can protect against MS, whereas exposure to the same infections later in life, predisposes to MS [25]. The hygiene hypothesis also partly explained the geographical distribution of MS, in that it is less common in tropical regions that are known to be endemic to certain microbial infections. In these areas, children tend to acquire infections very early in life [26, 27]. Similarly, MS incidence seems to rise in tropical regions [28] that have witnessed improved feasibility of vaccines and antibiotics and enhanced sanitary conditions which have led to decreased childhood infections [29–31]. However, some epidemiological observations such as the finding that the risk of MS in individuals who have never been exposed to EBV is 10 fold lower than in those who were exposed to childhood EBV infection [32], cannot be explained by the hygiene hypothesis.

2. Epstein-Barr virus (EBV)

EBV is a common human herpesvirus, infecting over 90% of the population worldwide [33]. Generally, EBV infection is considered to be one of the early asymptomatic childhood infections and in the vast majority of the infected individuals, the virus persists for life without causing disease. Bizarrely, if primary infection is delayed until adolescence, as commonly noted in developed countries, the virus can cause an acute self-limiting symptomatic infection known as infectious mononucleosis (IM) [34]. Importantly, EBV has oncogenic properties and in a very small percentage of individuals, the virus can induce life-threatening lymphoid and epithelial malignancies, accounting for approximately 150,000 deaths annually [35, 36].

EBV is transmitted from person to person through salivary exchange. However, the details of the early steps in EBV infection remain unclear. Two models have been proposed. In the first model, it is suggested that EBV initially infects tonsillar epithelial cells where it undergoes lytic replication with subsequent infection of B-lymphocytes. In the second model, it is suggested that EBV directly infects B-lymphocytes without the involvement of epithelial cells [37, 38]. Whatever the initial cellular target, one thing is fairly well-established; the cellular site of long-term EBV persistence is B-lymphocytes [39, 40]. These cells can be transformed and immortalized by EBV when grown in *in vitro* cultures, forming what are known as lymphoblastoid cell lines (LCLs). In LCLs, a number of viral latent products, namely 2 EBV encoded RNAs (EBER 1 and 2), 6 EBV nuclear antigens (EBNAs 1, 2, 3A, 3B, 3C and LP) and 3 EBV latent membrane proteins (LMPs 1, 2A and 2B) are expressed [33]. The expression of these latent products in infected cells is referred to as EBV latency III program and is typically observed in EBV associated post-transplant lymphomas [41] and in IM [42]. When EBERs, EBNA-1, LMP1 and LMP2 are expressed, it is known as latency II, typically seen in EBV associated Hodgkin's lymphoma. In latency I, only EBERs and EBNA-1 are expressed, as seen in Burkitt's lymphoma. In latently infected asymptomatic EBV carriers (>90% of the population), infected B cells express EBERs only [43]. Since no viral proteins are expressed in these cells, the virus can remain out of the radar of the host immune system. This strategy allows the virus to be dormant, but still dangerous. Moreover, the virus utilizes an array of viral encoded miRNAs to target immune associated mRNAs, aiding its escape from host defenses [44, 45]. Thus, EBV has evolved to be a master manipulator of the immune system, ensuring its persistence for the life of its host, even in the face of a competent immune system.

Beside the latent infection described above, a lytic infection can occasionally occur resulting in production of new virions. The expression of the immediate early lytic protein BZLF1 signals the beginning of the lytic cycle. Whether it is latent or lytic infection, an efficiently functioning immune system is essential to keep EBV infection under control and maintain a homeostatic virus-host relationship [46]. Thus, any disruption of the intricate connection between EBV and the immune system can lead to serious health conditions, for instance EBV-induced malignancies and some autoimmune disorders such as MS. Based on an accumulating body of evidence from epidemiological, serological and postmortem studies, it is now widely believed that EBV is associated, directly or indirectly in the pathogenesis of MS [20–22]. However, the details of how EBV induces or promotes an aberrant immune response against myelin self-antigens in MS remain unknown.

3. Epidemiological link between EBV and MS

A considerable amount of literature has been published on the link between the epidemiology of MS and EBV infection. Early reports consistently showed higher prevalence of EBV infection in MS patients compared to the general population [47, 48]. This difference was particularly pronounced in the pediatric cohort, where almost 100% of children with MS were EBV seropositive compared to 72% matched controls [49–52]. Consistent with these findings, MS risk was found to diminish in individuals who have never been exposed to EBV infection (the odds ratio of developing MS is 0.06 in a seronegative person compared to 13.5 in an EBV seropositive person). Furthermore, continuing to be EBV seronegative keeps MS risk to about

10-fold lower than those who seroconvert [53] and about 20-fold less than those with a history of IM, the primary symptomatic EBV infection [32]. These reports suggest that the risk of MS rises in EBV-seronegative individuals soon after they seroconvert as confirmed by a nested case–control study on 305 MS cases and 610 controls [54].

Interestingly, IM has a strikingly similar distribution to that of MS [55]. Moreover, females report IM symptoms earlier (more prolonged), more frequently, and with more severity than their male counterparts. Females also tend to have higher anti-EBV titers and are believed to mount stronger response against EBV [56, 57]. In demonstration of the correlation between IM and the risk of MS, a case–control study found that history of IM increases the risk of developing a CNS demyelinating disease, particularly in genetically susceptible individuals who are HLA-DRB1*1501 positive [58]. In support of these results, a meta-analysis of 14 case–control and longitudinal studies reported that history of IM significantly increased the risk of MS by over 2 folds [59]. Furthermore, this increased risk persists for at least 30 years post EBV infection [60], suggesting that symptomatic EBV infection manifested as IM may be a prerequisite to developing the autoimmune response associated with MS [61].

4. Serological link between EBV and MS

More evidence has been brought to light by serological studies investigating antibody response against EBV antigens in MS patients compared to that in controls. One of the most consist piece of evidence is the finding of elevated antibody titers against EBNA-1 antigen in the blood, both pre- and post-onset of the disease [62–65]. Indeed, individuals with clinically isolated syndromes (CIS) are more likely to develop definite MS when they experience elevated antibody response to EBNA-1 [66, 67]. Furthermore, serum levels of anti-EBV capsid antigen (VCA) together with anti-EBNA-1 IgG antibodies seem to also correlate with the risk of MS [68]. In an attempt to understand how the humoral response towards EBNA-1 impacts the risk of developing MS, it was shown that the levels of circulating IgG against certain EBNA-1 epitopes, particularly those derived from EBNA-1: 385–420 domain, interact with MS risk gene, the HLA genotype DRB1*15 in amplifying MS risk [69]. These findings point to similarities between how HLA molecules influence response to EBV antigens and how they are involved in inducing autoimmune response [70]. Additionally, the humoral response to EBV antigens, specifically anti-EBNA-1 IgG vary between different forms of MS, namely CIS, relapsing–remitting and progressive MS [71], suggesting that the level of these antibodies is not only predictive of MS onset, but also of disease progression. However, it remains debatable whether the humoral level can correlate with markers of disease progression such as volumes of T2 MRI lesions, reflective of demyelinative disease activity and scores of Expanded Disability Status Scale (EDSS), reflective of the progression of physical disability [71–76]. Despite some of these inconsistencies in the serological link between EBV infection and MS, studies agree on the fact that serum antibody titers to EBNA-1 increase prior to developing MS, and hence predictive of MS. In other words, it seems that EBV acts early in provoking an immune (humoral) response towards promoting the onset of MS [77]. However, it is safe to argue that EBV may be a cofactor contributing with other factors, such as genetic susceptibility and vitamin D levels, to the pathogenesis of MS [78, 79].

5. Cellular immune response to EBV in MS

Forty years ago, it was shown that peripheral blood mononuclear cells (PBMCs) taken from patients with active MS, spontaneously transformed into LCLs in *in vitro* culture more readily than PBMCs taken from healthy controls or patients with inactive MS [80]. These spontaneously immortalized LCLs were of B-cell origin and expressed EBV antigens, including VCA and EBNAs [80]. So, why do PBMCs from active MS patients transform more readily compared to those from healthy controls? One possible explanation is that the immune response to EBV in MS patients is less effective compared to healthy EBV seropositive individuals. Indeed, data from a number of different studies indicates that the T-cell response to EBV is aberrantly regulated in MS patients and it varies at different stages of the disease [81–83]. $CD8^+$ T cells in the blood of MS patients with inactive disease, have been shown to express the immune inhibitory molecule, programmed death 1 (PD-1), making these cells less efficient in eliminating EBV infected cells [84]. This $CD8^+$ T cell exhaustion is believed to be a common feature in many chronic viral infections [85–87], and could explain the conflicting results in EBV viral load detected in MS patients. Thus, the stage of the disease and the level of T cell exhaustion could account for the higher viral load reported in some studies [88, 89], whilst others showed no statistical difference between MS and controls [89–91]. Further support for an aberrant anti-viral immune response in MS comes from the observations that MS patients appear to be at increased risk of acquiring certain viral infections such as influenza [92, 93].

A more recent study investigated B cell transformation of PBMCs taken from 21 MS patients and 21 healthy controls [94]. In order to minimize the effect of T cell control of EBV, which may vary from person to person, T cell activity in all PBMCs cultures was inhibited using cyclosporine A. Cultures obtained from MS patients resulted in significantly higher frequency of B cell transformation compared to healthy controls [94]. Whether this was due to MS patients having a higher frequency of circulating EBV infected cells, or due to higher frequency of viral lytic replication occurring in MS patients is not clear.

There have also been some attempts to examine differences in the cell-mediated immune response against EBV and its antigens in the blood and cerebrospinal fluid (CSF) of MS patients [95, 96]. However, these investigations have also yielded inconsistent results. Whilst some have reported an increase in frequency of both intrathecal EBV reactive $CD4^+$ and $CD8^+$ T cells in MS [96], others have found that only $CD8^+$ T cells and not $CD4^+$ T cells are increased compared to controls [95]. Moreover, intrathecal $CD4^+$ and $CD8^+$ T cells from MS failed to react to a number of common autoantigens suspected to be targets of immune response in MS [97]. Thus, the identity of the target antigen for the autoreactive T cells remains elusive. A very recent study has reported that intrathecal $CD4^+$ T cells from HLA-DRB3 positive MS patients reacted with GDP-L-fucose synthase, an enzyme frequently expressed in human cells as well as in bacteria commonly present in the gastrointestinal track of MS patients [98]. This tantalizing finding warrants further investigations to determine if gut bacterial GDP-L-fucose synthase is indeed the primary trigger for the activation of autoreactive T-cells that subsequently migrate to the brain and lead to demyelination. It is plausible that EBV could also trigger autoreactive T-cells by molecularly mimicry [99–101]. In this context, certain epitopes of EBNA-1, EBNA-3A and LMP2 have been shown to be targets of $CD8^+$ T cell responses and to cross-react with self-antigens associated with MS pathogenesis [102–104]. However, current evidence fails to clearly explain how cell-mediated immune responses to EBV antigens may lead to MS.

6. Direct demonstration of the presence of EBV in MS brains

Compared to the blood and CSF, access to brain tissues, particularly fresh tissues from MS patients has been difficult and limited. In spite of this, a number of studies have examined brain tissues to explore the link between EBV and the pathogenesis of MS. Most of these investigations have been conducted on formalin-fixed, paraffin-embedded post-mortem tissues. Arguably, these studies have generated the strongest and most convincing data implicating EBV in the development of MS. Initial attempts aimed at directly demonstrating if EBV was present in MS lesions or not, reported either negative results or did not see any difference in EBV positivity between MS and control tissues [105, 106]. A subsequent study however, reported the presence of EBV in 21/22 MS, but not in non-MS inflammatory neurological conditions [107]. The virus was localized to B cells and plasma cells, most notably in the meninges and perivascular infiltrates of active lesions. Additionally, infected cells were found to express a number of viral antigens, latent and lytic [107], making them a potential target of $CD8^+$ T cells and triggering an inflammatory environment in the CNS [82]. Although these findings were confirmed by some subsequent studies [108, 109], others reported absence of EBV infection in the MS brain [110–112]. It was argued that the discrepancies in the findings would be due to many different variables, including differences in the tissue samples examined, variation in tissue preservation and processing, type of fixatives and length of fixation, and the sensitivity and specificity of methods used for EBV detection [113]. Moreover, owing to the great heterogeneity of the brain, the molecular and cellular environment of one region does not necessarily represent another adjacent region, even in the same tissue block [113, 114]. Thus, the absence of EBV in one region of the brain, cannot be interpreted to mean that the virus is absent from all parts of the brain. Keeping some of these variables in mind, we recently conducted an extensive study examining the potential involvement of EBV in MS pathogenesis [115]. We analyzed over 1000 samples from MS cases and non-MS controls using our highly sensitive EBER-*in situ* hybridization, PCR, and immunohistochemistry methodologies [115]. Our findings indicated that EBV was present in most (90%) cases of MS and the virus could be detected in multiple tissue samples from each case. Surprisingly, we found EBV not only in B-cells, but also in astrocytes and some microglial cells. Significantly, the virus was transcriptionally active in these cells and expressed EBNA-1, and to a lesser extent the early lytic cycle protein BZLF1. Taken together, these findings support a role for EBV in the pathogenesis of MS.

7. Proposed model of EBV involvement in MS pathology

The data demonstrating the presence of EBV directly in the brain of MS cases is fairly robust and convincing evidence in support of a role for EBV in the pathogenesis of MS. However, the presence of the virus in the brain cannot be simply interpreted to imply causality. Although it is possible that EBV infection could be a consequence of MS pathology, the observation that EBV seronegative individuals have an almost zero risk of developing MS is strong and compelling evidence supporting a role for EBV in initiating MS. Ironically, although it is believed that T-cells orchestrate and lead the pathogenesis of MS, treatment strategies that have been shown to be most effective in controlling disease activity, involve depleting B-cells [22, 116]. Moreover, depleting memory B-cells, the very cells that harbor EBV, appears to be the most effective [117]. How can these apparently contradictory findings be reconciled? We propose that EBV infected memory B-cells act as antigen presenting cells (APC), resulting in the activation of helper T-cells, which in individuals carrying certain HLA haplotypes, activate autoreactive B and T-cells targeting antigens expressed on oligodendrocytes [102, 118]. In this model (**Figure 1**), disturbances in the integrity of the blood brain barrier (BBB) allows EBV carrying memory B-cells to cross into the CNS, triggering a cascade of events including, attraction of autoreactive B and T-cells, triggering pro-inflammatory cytokines and microglial activation [118–120]. While most of the EBV infected B-cells infiltrating into the brain remain latently infected, a small percentage are triggered to undergo lytic replication [121, 122, 107], which could explain how CNS resident astrocytes and microglial cells get infected [115]. Infection of astrocytes can be reconciled by the fact that, like B-cells, they also express CD21, the receptor for EBV [123]. Astrocytes are the most abundant cells in the CNS, constituting around 30% of the total cells. They play an important role in a number of homeostatic and neuroinflammatory processes within the CNS, including axon guidance, synaptic transmission and controlling BBB [124, 125]. An accumulating body of data now indicates that activated astrocytes also play a central role in neurodegenerative diseases such as MS [124–126]. Since astrocytes interact with blood vessels to form the BBB, any functional impact on these cells could also increase BBB permeability and exacerbate infiltration of peripheral immune cells into the CNS [120, 125, 127]. This could explain the characteristic perivascular cuffing and presence of inflammatory aggregates resembling germinal center (GC)-like structures commonly observed in the CNS in viral infections [22, 128]. Although the precise role of these tertiary lymphoid aggregates remains unknown, it is likely that they play a key role

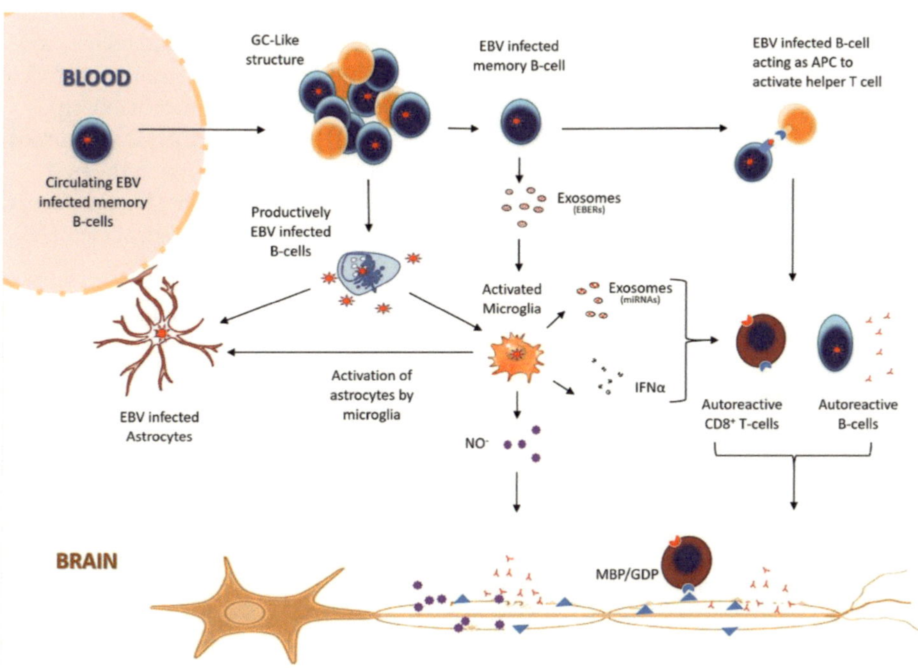

Figure 1.
Model for EBV involvement in MS pathology. The pathogenesis of MS is no doubt very complex. This is a simplified outline of a potential model to explain some of the experimental findings linking EBV to MS. EBV persists in memory B-cells in peripheral circulation [39, 40] and in healthy seropositive individuals, they are tightly regulated by the immune system. In individuals genetically predisposed to MS, these cells cross the BBB and enter the CNS where they trigger an inflammatory response leading to the formation of GC-like structures [128, 129]. Most of the infected cells remain latently infected with limited viral gene expression [107, 108]. These infected cells could function as APC for the activation of helper T-cells [118] which in individuals carrying certain HLA haplotypes [89, 132], leads to the activation of autoreactive B and T-cells that recognize both EBV and self-antigens [99, 101, 118]. A small proportion of EBV infected memory B-cells, upon differentiation into plasma cells, initiate EBV replicative cycle [121, 122]. The new virions produced, infect other susceptible cells, including astrocytes and microglia [115, 123]. Microglia and astrocytes are two main types of cells typically providing a protective role against viral infection. In their activated form, they release various pro-inflammatory cytokines and immune mediators that activate the immune system to resolve the infection [125, 133]. In MS, these chronically activated cells switch from being neuroprotective to neurotoxic [133, 134]. Additionally, proinflammatory microglia can also induce activation of astrocytes, which can impact not only the BBB but also contribute to neurotoxicity [125, 126]. The combined effects of these multiple events result in MS pathology.

in the immune response to CNS injury [129]. In contrast to previously held views, studies now indicate that B-cell differentiation and clonal expansion typically known to occur in secondary lymphoid organs, can also occur in the CNS [130]. This finding also provides an explanation for the source of oligoclonal immunoglobulin bands present in the CSF of most patients with MS. In MS, these GC-like aggregates, triggered by EBV infection of the brain, could be responsible for recruiting, activating and sustaining B and T-cells [119, 118] that inadvertently react to auto-antigens, such as myelin basic protein (MBP) and GDP-L-fucose synthase, expressed on oligodendrocytes (**Figure 1**) [98, 99, 101]. Moreover, cellular and viral components such miRNAs and EBERs, secreted in exosomes could also promote inflammatory and pathological changes that contribute to CNS injury in MS [108, 131].

8. Conclusion

The pathogenesis of MS appears to be a complex process, where both genetic and environmental risk factors interplay to promote the development of the disease. The evidence implicating EBV as a central player in MS development is substantial. For some critics, these pieces of evidence are still not sufficient to charge EBV as the mastermind behind the pathogenesis of MS. A very recent study by Pender and colleagues goes some way to proving the etiological association [135]. The study demonstrated that treating MS patients with autologous EBV-specific T cell therapy can improve symptoms and quality of life in most patients [135]. The only absolute and unequivocal proof that EBV is central to the development of MS, is to prevent EBV infection in the first place by vaccination and then see if the incidence of MS declines. Although a number of vaccine candidates have been tested, none have yet been approved for clinical use [136].

Acknowledgements

This work was supported by UAEU grants (31 M376 & 31 R135) awarded to GK and PhD Scholarship awarded to AH from UAE University.

Conflict of interest

The authors have no conflict of interest.

Author details

Gulfaraz Khan* and Asma Hassani
Department of Microbiology and Immunology, College of Medicine and Health Sciences, Tawam Hospital Campus, United Arab Emirates University, Al Ain, UAE

*Address all correspondence to: g_khan@uaeu.ac.ae

References

[1] Compston A, Coles A. Multiple sclerosis. Lancet. 2008;**372**:1502-1517

[2] Baranzini SE, Oksenberg JR. The genetics of multiple sclerosis: From 0 to 200 in 50 years. Trends in Genetics. 2017;**33**:960-970

[3] Gourraud P-A, Harbo HF, Hauser SL, et al. The genetics of multiple sclerosis: An up-to-date review. Immunological Reviews. 2012;**248**:87-103

[4] Dilokthornsakul P, Valuck RJ, Nair KV, et al. Multiple sclerosis prevalence in the United States commercially insured population. Neurology. 2016;**86**:1014-1021

[5] Rosati G. The prevalence of multiple sclerosis in the world: An update. Neurological Sciences. 2001;**22**:117-139

[6] Wallin MT, Culpepper WJ, Coffman P, et al. The gulf war era multiple sclerosis cohort: Age and incidence rates by race, sex and service. Brain. 2012;**135**:1778-1785

[7] Langer-Gould A, Brara SM, Beaber BE, et al. Incidence of multiple sclerosis in multiple racial and ethnic groups. Neurology. 2013;**80**:1734-1739

[8] Compston A. The genetic epidemiology of multiple sclerosis. Philosophical Transactions of the Royal Society of London. Series B, Biological Sciences. 1999;**354**:1623-1634

[9] Hansen T, Skytthe A, Stenager E, et al. Risk for multiple sclerosis in dizygotic and monozygotic twins. Multiple Sclerosis. 2005;**11**:500-503

[10] Wade BJ. Spatial analysis of global prevalence of multiple sclerosis suggests need for an updated prevalence scale. Multiple Sclerosis International. 2014;**2014**:124578

[11] Melcon MO, Correale J, Melcon CM. Is it time for a new global classification of multiple sclerosis? Journal of the Neurological Sciences. 2014;**344**:171-181

[12] Koch-Henriksen N, Sørensen PS. The changing demographic pattern of multiple sclerosis epidemiology. Lancet Neurology. 2010;**9**:520-532

[13] Berg-Hansen P, Celius EG. Socio-economic factors and immigrant population studies of multiple sclerosis. Acta Neurologica Scandinavica. 2015;**132**:37-41

[14] Nasr Z, Majed M, Rostami A, et al. Prevalence of multiple sclerosis in Iranian emigrants: Review of the evidence. Neurological Sciences. 2016;**37**:1759-1763

[15] Ahlgren C, Lycke J, Odén A, et al. High risk of MS in Iranian immigrants in Gothenburg, Sweden. Multiple Sclerosis. 2010;**16**:1079-1082

[16] Berg-Hansen P, Moen SM, Sandvik L, et al. Prevalence of multiple sclerosis among immigrants in Norway. Multiple Sclerosis. 2015;**21**:695-702

[17] Milo R, Kahana E. Multiple sclerosis: Geoepidemiology, genetics and the environment. Autoimmunity Reviews. 2010;**9**:A387-A394

[18] McLeod JG, Hammond SR, Kurtzke JF. Migration and multiple sclerosis in immigrants to Australia from United Kingdom and Ireland: A reassessment. I. Risk of MS by age at immigration. Journal of Neurology. 2011;**258**:1140-1149

[19] Ascherio A, Munger KL. Environmental risk factors for multiple sclerosis. Part II: Noninfectious factors. Annals of Neurology. 2007;**61**:504-513

[20] Ascherio A, Munger KL, Lünemann JD. The initiation and

prevention of multiple sclerosis. Nature Reviews. Neurology. 2012;**8**:602-612

[21] Correale J, Gaitán MI. Multiple sclerosis and environmental factors: The role of vitamin D, parasites, and Epstein-Barr virus infection. Acta Neurologica Scandinavica. 2015;**132**:46-55

[22] Reich DS, Lucchinetti CF, Calabresi PA. Multiple sclerosis. The New England Journal of Medicine. 2018;**378**:169-180

[23] Belbasis L, Bellou V, Evangelou E, et al. Environmental risk factors and multiple sclerosis: An umbrella review of systematic reviews and meta-analyses. Lancet Neurology. 2015;**14**:263-273

[24] Wallin MT, Heltberg A, Kurtzke JF. Multiple sclerosis in the Faroe Islands. 8. Notifiable diseases. Acta Neurologica Scandinavica. 2010;**122**:102-109

[25] Hughes A-M, Lucas RM, McMichael AJ, et al. Early-life hygiene-related factors affect risk of central nervous system demyelination and asthma differentially. Clinical and Experimental Immunology. 2013;**172**:466-474

[26] Gustavsen MW, Page CM, Moen SM, et al. Environmental exposures and the risk of multiple sclerosis investigated in a Norwegian case-control study. BMC Neurology. 2014;**14**:196

[27] Pedrini MJF, Seewann A, Bennett KA, et al. Helicobacter pylori infection as a protective factor against multiple sclerosis risk in females. Journal of Neurology, Neurosurgery, and Psychiatry. 2015;**86**:603-607

[28] Eskandarieh S, Heydarpour P, Minagar A, et al. Multiple sclerosis epidemiology in East Asia, South East Asia and South Asia: A systematic review. Neuroepidemiology. 2016;**46**:209-221

[29] Wendel-Haga M, Celius EG. Is the hygiene hypothesis relevant for the risk of multiple sclerosis? Acta Neurologica Scandinavica. 2017;**136**(Suppl 201):26-30

[30] Libbey JE, Cusick MF, Fujinami RS. Role of pathogens in multiple sclerosis. International Reviews of Immunology. 2014;**33**:266-283

[31] Lim Y, Romano N, Colin N, et al. Intestinal parasitic infections amongst orang Asli (indigenous) in Malaysia: Has socioeconomic development alleviated the problem? Tropical Biomedicine. 2009;**26**:110-122

[32] Ascherio A, Munger KL. 99th Dahlem conference on infection, inflammation and chronic inflammatory disorders: Epstein-Barr virus and multiple sclerosis: Epidemiological evidence. Clinical and Experimental Immunology. 2010;**160**:120-124

[33] Young LS, Yap LF, Murray PG. Epstein-Barr virus: More than 50 years old and still providing surprises. Nature Reviews. Cancer. 2016;**16**:789-802

[34] Dunmire SK, Verghese PS, Balfour HH. Primary Epstein-Barr virus infection. Journal of Clinical Virology. 2018;**102**:84-92

[35] Niedobitek G, Meru N, Delecluse HJ. Epstein-Barr virus infection and human malignancies. International Journal of Experimental Pathology. 2001;**82**:149-170

[36] Khan G, Hashim MJ. Global burden of deaths from Epstein-Barr virus attributable malignancies 1990-2010. Infectious Agents and Cancer. 2014;**9**:38

[37] Young LS, Rickinson AB. Epstein-Barr virus: 40 years on. Nature Reviews. Cancer. 2004;**4**:757-768

[38] Thorley-Lawson DA, Miyashita EM, Khan G. Epstein-Barr virus and the

B cell: That's all it takes. Trends in Microbiology. 1996;**4**:204-208

[39] Babcock GJ, Decker LL, Volk M, et al. EBV persistence in memory B cells in vivo. Immunity. 1998;**9**:395-404

[40] Khan G, Miyashita EM, Yang B, et al. Is EBV persistence in vivo a model for B cell homeostasis? Immunity. 1996;**5**:173-179

[41] Brink AA, Dukers DF, van den Brule AJ, et al. Presence of Epstein-Barr virus latency type III at the single cell level in post-transplantation lymphoproliferative disorders and AIDS related lymphomas. Journal of Clinical Pathology. 1997;**50**:911-918

[42] Tierney RJ, Steven N, Young LS, et al. Epstein-Barr virus latency in blood mononuclear cells: Analysis of viral gene transcription during primary infection and in the carrier state. Journal of Virology. 1994;**68**:7374-7385

[43] Thorley-Lawson DA. EBV persistence–Introducing the virus. Current Topics in Microbiology and Immunology. 2015;**390**:151-209

[44] Skalsky RL, Cullen BR. EBV noncoding RNAs. Current Topics in Microbiology and Immunology. 2015;**391**:181-217

[45] Kaul V, Weinberg KI, Boyd SD, et al. Dynamics of viral and host immune cell microRNA expression during acute infectious mononucleosis. Frontiers in Microbiology. 2017;**8**:2666

[46] Münz C. Epstein Barr virus–A tumor virus that needs cytotoxic lymphocytes to persist asymptomatically. Current Opinion in Virology. 2016;**20**:34-39

[47] Sumaya CV, Myers LW, Ellison GW. Epstein-Barr virus antibodies in multiple sclerosis. Archives of Neurology. 1980;**37**:94-96

[48] Sumaya CV, Myers LW, Ellison GW, et al. Increased prevalence and titer of Epstein-Barr virus antibodies in patients with multiple sclerosis. Annals of Neurology. 1985;**17**:371-377

[49] Pohl D, Krone B, Rostasy K, et al. High seroprevalence of Epstein-Barr virus in children with multiple sclerosis. Neurology. 2006;**67**:2063-2065

[50] Banwell B, Krupp L, Kennedy J, et al. Clinical features and viral serologies in children with multiple sclerosis: A multinational observational study. Lancet Neurology. 2007;**6**:773-781

[51] Alotaibi S, Kennedy J, Tellier R, et al. Epstein-Barr virus in pediatric multiple sclerosis. JAMA. 2004;**291**:1875-1879

[52] Waubant E, Mowry EM, Krupp L, et al. Common viruses associated with lower pediatric multiple sclerosis risk. Neurology. 2011;**76**:1989-1995

[53] Ascherio A, Munch M. Epstein-Barr virus and multiple sclerosis. Epidemiology. 2000;**11**:220-224

[54] Levin LI, Munger KL, O'Reilly EJ, et al. Primary infection with the Epstein-Barr virus and risk of multiple sclerosis. Annals of Neurology. 2010;**67**:824-830

[55] Warner HB, Carp RI. Multiple sclerosis and Epstein-Barr virus. Lancet. 1981;**2**:1290

[56] Sawyer RN, Evans AS, Niederman JC, et al. Prospective studies of a group of Yale University freshmen. I. Occurrence of infectious mononucleosis. The Journal of Infectious Diseases. 1971;**123**:263-270

[57] Macsween KF, Higgins CD, McAulay KA, et al. Infectious mononucleosis in university students in the United Kingdom: Evaluation of the clinical features and consequences of the disease. Clinical Infectious Diseases. 2010;**50**:699-706

[58] Lucas RM, Ponsonby A-L, Dear K, et al. Current and past Epstein-Barr virus infection in risk of initial CNS demyelination. Neurology. 2011;77:371-379

[59] Thacker EL, Mirzaei F, Ascherio A. Infectious mononucleosis and risk for multiple sclerosis: A meta-analysis. Annals of Neurology. 2006;**59**:499-503

[60] Nielsen TR, Rostgaard K, Nielsen NM, et al. Multiple sclerosis after infectious mononucleosis. Archives of Neurology. 2007;**64**:72-75

[61] Haahr S, Koch-Henriksen N, Møller-Larsen A, et al. Increased risk of multiple sclerosis after late Epstein-Barr virus infection: A historical prospective study. Multiple Sclerosis. 1995;**1**:73-77

[62] Levin LI, Munger KL, Rubertone MV, et al. Temporal relationship between elevation of Epstein-Barr virus antibody titers and initial onset of neurological symptoms in multiple sclerosis. JAMA. 2005;**293**:2496-2500

[63] Sundström P, Juto P, Wadell G, et al. An altered immune response to Epstein-Barr virus in multiple sclerosis: A prospective study. Neurology. 2004;**62**:2277-2282

[64] DeLorenze GN, Munger KL, Lennette ET, et al. Epstein-Barr virus and multiple sclerosis: Evidence of association from a prospective study with long-term follow-up. Archives of Neurology. 2006;**63**:839-844

[65] Comabella M, Montalban X, Horga A, et al. Antiviral immune response in patients with multiple sclerosis and healthy siblings. Multiple Sclerosis. 2010;**16**:355-358

[66] Lünemann JD, Tintoré M, Messmer B, et al. Elevated Epstein-Barr virus-encoded nuclear antigen-1 immune responses predict conversion to multiple sclerosis. Annals of Neurology. 2010;**67**:159-169

[67] Schlemm L, Giess RM, Rasche L, et al. Fine specificity of the antibody response to Epstein-Barr nuclear antigen-2 and other Epstein-Barr virus proteins in patients with clinically isolated syndrome: A peptide microarray-based case-control study. Journal of Neuroimmunology. 2016;**297**:56-62

[68] Ascherio A, Munger KL, Lennette ET, et al. Epstein-Barr virus antibodies and risk of multiple sclerosis: A prospective study. JAMA. 2001;**286**:3083-3088

[69] Sundqvist E, Sundström P, Lindén M, et al. Epstein-Barr virus and multiple sclerosis: Interaction with HLA. Genes and Immunity. 2012;**13**:14-20

[70] Rubicz R, Yolken R, Drigalenko E, et al. A genome-wide integrative genomic study localizes genetic factors influencing antibodies against Epstein-Barr virus nuclear antigen 1 (EBNA-1). PLoS Genetics. 2013;**9**:e1003147

[71] Farrell RA, Antony D, Wall GR, et al. Humoral immune response to EBV in multiple sclerosis is associated with disease activity on MRI. Neurology. 2009;**73**:32-38

[72] Almohmeed YH, Avenell A, Aucott L, et al. Systematic review and meta-analysis of the sero-epidemiological association between Epstein Barr virus and multiple sclerosis. PLoS One. 2013;**8**:e61110

[73] Zivadinov R, Cerza N, Hagemeier J, et al. Humoral response to EBV is associated with cortical atrophy and lesion burden in patients with MS. Neurology Neuroimmunology & Neuroinflammation. 2016;**3**:e190

[74] Wandinger K, Jabs W, Siekhaus A, et al. Association between clinical

disease activity and Epstein-Barr virus reactivation in MS. Neurology. 2000;**55**:178-184

[75] Buljevac D, van Doornum GJJ, Flach HZ, et al. Epstein-Barr virus and disease activity in multiple sclerosis. Journal of Neurology, Neurosurgery, and Psychiatry. 2005;**76**:1377-1381

[76] Gieß RM, Pfuhl C, Behrens JR, et al. Epstein-Barr virus antibodies in serum and DNA load in saliva are not associated with radiological or clinical disease activity in patients with early multiple sclerosis. PLoS One. 2017;**12**:e0175279

[77] Kakalacheva K, Regenass S, Wiesmayr S, et al. Infectious mononucleosis triggers generation of IgG auto-antibodies against native myelin oligodendrocyte glycoprotein. Viruses. 2016;**8**. DOI: 10.3390/v8020051

[78] Wergeland S, Myhr K-M, Løken-Amsrud KI, et al. Vitamin D, HLA-DRB1 and Epstein-Barr virus antibody levels in a prospective cohort of multiple sclerosis patients. European Journal of Neurology. 2016;**23**:1064-1070

[79] Rolf L, Muris A-H, Mathias A, et al. Exploring the effect of vitamin D3 supplementation on the anti-EBV antibody response in relapsing-remitting multiple sclerosis. Multiple Sclerosis. 2018;**24**:1280-1287

[80] Fraser KB, Haire M, Millar JH, et al. Increased tendency to spontaneous in-vitro lymphocyte transformation in clinically active multiple sclerosis. Lancet. 1979;**2**:175-176

[81] Jilek S, Schluep M, Harari A, et al. HLA-B7-restricted EBV-specific CD8+ T cells are dysregulated in multiple sclerosis. Journal of Immunology. 2012;**188**:4671-4680

[82] Angelini DF, Serafini B, Piras E, et al. Increased CD8+ T cell response to Epstein-Barr virus lytic antigens in the active phase of multiple sclerosis. PLoS Pathogens. 2013;**9**:e1003220

[83] Pender MP, Csurhes PA, Burrows JM, et al. Defective T-cell control of Epstein-Barr virus infection in multiple sclerosis. Clinical & Translational Immunology. 2017;**6**:e126

[84] Cencioni MT, Magliozzi R, Nicholas R, et al. Programmed death 1 is highly expressed on CD8+ CD57+ T cells in patients with stable multiple sclerosis and inhibits their cytotoxic response to Epstein-Barr virus. Immunology. 2017;**152**:660-676

[85] Day CL, Kaufmann DE, Kiepiela P, et al. PD-1 expression on HIV-specific T cells is associated with T-cell exhaustion and disease progression. Nature. 2006;**443**:350-354

[86] Barber DL, Wherry EJ, Masopust D, et al. Restoring function in exhausted CD8 T cells during chronic viral infection. Nature. 2006;**439**:682-687

[87] Wherry EJ. T cell exhaustion. Nature Immunology. 2011;**12**:492-499

[88] Wagner H-J, Munger KL, Ascherio A. Plasma viral load of Epstein-Barr virus and risk of multiple sclerosis. European Journal of Neurology. 2004;**11**:833-834

[89] Agostini S, Mancuso R, Guerini FR, et al. HLA alleles modulate EBV viral load in multiple sclerosis. Journal of Translational Medicine. 2018;**16**:80

[90] Lindsey JW, Hatfield LM, Crawford MP, et al. Quantitative PCR for Epstein-Barr virus DNA and RNA in multiple sclerosis. Multiple Sclerosis. 2009;**15**:153-158

[91] Holden DW, Gold J, Hawkes CH, et al. Epstein Barr virus shedding in multiple sclerosis: Similar frequencies of EBV in saliva across separate patient

cohorts. Multiple Sclerosis and Related Disorders. 2018;**25**:197-199

[92] Marrie RA, Elliott L, Marriott J, et al. Dramatically changing rates and reasons for hospitalization in multiple sclerosis. Neurology. 2014;**83**:929-937

[93] Glenn JD, Smith MD, Xue P, et al. CNS-targeted autoimmunity leads to increased influenza mortality in mice. Journal of Experimental Medicine. 2017;**214**:297-307

[94] Tørring C, Andreasen C, Gehr N, et al. Higher incidence of Epstein-Barr virus-induced lymphocyte transformation in multiple sclerosis. Acta Neurologica Scandinavica. 2014;**130**:90-96

[95] Lossius A, Johansen JN, Vartdal F, et al. High-throughput sequencing of TCR repertoires in multiple sclerosis reveals intrathecal enrichment of EBV-reactive CD8+ T cells. European Journal of Immunology. 2014;**44**:3439-3452

[96] van Nierop GP, Mautner J, Mitterreiter JG, et al. Intrathecal CD8 T-cells of multiple sclerosis patients recognize lytic Epstein-Barr virus proteins. Multiple Sclerosis. 2016;**22**:279-291

[97] van Nierop GP, Janssen M, Mitterreiter JG, et al. Intrathecal CD4(+) and CD8(+) T-cell responses to endogenously synthesized candidate disease-associated human autoantigens in multiple sclerosis patients. European Journal of Immunology. 2016;**46**:347-353

[98] Planas R, Santos R, Tomas-Ojer P, et al. GDP-l-fucose synthase is a CD4+ T cell–specific autoantigen in DRB3*02:02 patients with multiple sclerosis. Science Translational Medicine. 2018;**10**:eaat4301

[99] Wekerle H, Hohlfeld R. Molecular mimicry in multiple sclerosis. The New England Journal of Medicine. 2003;**349**:185-186

[100] Wherry EJ, Kurachi M. Molecular and cellular insights into T cell exhaustion. Nature Reviews. Immunology. 2015;**15**:486-499

[101] Geginat J, Paroni M, Pagani M, et al. The enigmatic role of viruses in multiple sclerosis: Molecular mimicry or disturbed immune surveillance? Trends in Immunology. 2017;**38**:498-512

[102] Lünemann JD, Jelcić I, Roberts S, et al. EBNA1-specific T cells from patients with multiple sclerosis cross react with myelin antigens and co-produce IFN-gamma and IL-2. The Journal of Experimental Medicine. 2008;**205**:1763-1773

[103] Cepok S, Zhou D, Srivastava R, et al. Identification of Epstein-Barr virus proteins as putative targets of the immune response in multiple sclerosis. The Journal of Clinical Investigation. 2005;**115**:1352-1360

[104] Lünemann JD, Edwards N, Muraro PA, et al. Increased frequency and broadened specificity of latent EBV nuclear antigen-1-specific T cells in multiple sclerosis. Brain. 2006;**129**:1493-1506

[105] Hilton DA, Love S, Fletcher A, et al. Absence of Epstein-Barr virus RNA in multiple sclerosis as assessed by in situ hybridisation. Journal of Neurology, Neurosurgery, and Psychiatry. 1994;**57**:975-976

[106] Opsahl ML, Kennedy PGE. An attempt to investigate the presence of Epstein Barr virus in multiple sclerosis and normal control brain tissue. Journal of Neurology. 2007;**254**:425-430

[107] Serafini B, Rosicarelli B, Franciotta D, et al. Dysregulated Epstein-Barr virus infection in the multiple sclerosis brain. The

Journal of Experimental Medicine. 2007;**204**:2899-2912

[108] Tzartos JS, Khan G, Vossenkamper A, et al. Association of innate immune activation with latent Epstein-Barr virus in active MS lesions. Neurology. 2012;**78**:15-23

[109] Magliozzi R, Serafini B, Rosicarelli B, et al. B-cell enrichment and Epstein-Barr virus infection in inflammatory cortical lesions in secondary progressive multiple sclerosis. Journal of Neuropathology and Experimental Neurology. 2013;**72**:29-41

[110] Willis SN, Stadelmann C, Rodig SJ, et al. Epstein-Barr virus infection is not a characteristic feature of multiple sclerosis brain. Brain. 2009;**132**:3318-3328

[111] Peferoen LAN, Lamers F, Lodder LNR, et al. Epstein Barr virus is not a characteristic feature in the central nervous system in established multiple sclerosis. Brain. 2010;**133**:e137

[112] Sargsyan SA, Shearer AJ, Ritchie AM, et al. Absence of Epstein-Barr virus in the brain and CSF of patients with multiple sclerosis. Neurology. 2010;**74**:1127-1135

[113] Lassmann H, Niedobitek G, Aloisi F, et al. Epstein-Barr virus in the multiple sclerosis brain: A controversial issue–Report on a focused workshop held in the Centre for Brain Research of the Medical University of Vienna, Austria. Brain. 2011;**134**:2772-2786

[114] Aloisi F, Serafini B, Magliozzi R, et al. Detection of Epstein-Barr virus and B-cell follicles in the multiple sclerosis brain: What you find depends on how and where you look. Brain. 2010;**133**:e157

[115] Hassani A, Corboy JR, Al-Salam S, et al. Epstein-Barr virus is present in the brain of most cases of multiple sclerosis and may engage more than just B cells. PLoS One. 2018;**13**:e0192109

[116] Naegelin Y, Naegelin P, von Felten S, et al. Association of rituximab treatment with disability progression among patients with secondary progressive multiple sclerosis. JAMA Neurology. 2019. DOI: 10.1001/jamaneurol.2018.4239

[117] Baker D, Marta M, Pryce G, et al. Memory B cells are major targets for effective immunotherapy in relapsing multiple sclerosis. eBioMedicine. 2017;**16**:41-50

[118] Jelcic I, Al Nimer F, Wang J, et al. Memory B cells activate brain-homing, autoreactive CD4+ T cells in multiple sclerosis. Cell. 2018;**175**:85-100. e23

[119] Michel L, Touil H, Pikor NB, et al. B Cells in the multiple sclerosis central nervous system: Trafficking and contribution to CNS-compartmentalized Inflammation. Frontiers in Immunology. 2015;**6**. DOI: 10.3389/fimmu.2015.00636

[120] Blauth K, Owens GP, Bennett JL. The ins and outs of B cells in multiple sclerosis. Frontiers in Immunology. 2015;**6**. DOI: 10.3389/fimmu.2015.00565

[121] Laichalk LL, Thorley-Lawson DA. Terminal differentiation into plasma cells initiates the replicative cycle of Epstein-Barr virus In vivo. Journal of Virology. 2005;**79**:1296-1307

[122] Moreno MA, Or-Geva N, Aftab BT, et al. Molecular signature of Epstein-Barr virus infection in MS brain lesions. Neurology–Neuroimmunology Neuroinflammation. 2018;**5**:e466

[123] Gasque P, Chan P, Mauger C, et al. Identification and characterization of complement C3 receptors on human astrocytes. The Journal of Immunology. 1996;**156**:2247-2255

[124] Sofroniew MV, Vinters HV. Astrocytes: Biology and pathology. Acta Neuropathologica. 2010;**119**:7-35

[125] Liddelow SA, Barres BA. Reactive astrocytes: Production, function, and therapeutic potential. Immunity. 2017;**46**:957-967

[126] Liddelow SA, Guttenplan KA, Clarke LE, et al. Neurotoxic reactive astrocytes are induced by activated microglia. Nature. 2017;**541**:481-487

[127] Sankowski R, Mader S, Valdés-Ferrer SI. Systemic inflammation and the brain: Novel roles of genetic, molecular, and environmental cues as drivers of neurodegeneration. Frontiers in Cellular Neuroscience. 2015;**9**. DOI: 10.3389/fncel.2015.00028

[128] Aloisi F, Pujol-Borrell R. Lymphoid neogenesis in chronic inflammatory diseases. Nature Reviews. Immunology. 2006;**6**:205-217

[129] Pikor NB, Prat A, Bar-Or A, et al. Meningeal tertiary lymphoid tissues and multiple sclerosis: A gathering place for diverse types of immune cells during CNS autoimmunity. Frontiers in Immunology. 2016;**6**. DOI: 10.3389/fimmu.2015.00657

[130] Corcione A, Casazza S, Ferretti E, et al. Recapitulation of B cell differentiation in the central nervous system of patients with multiple sclerosis. PNAS. 2004;**101**:11064-11069

[131] Ahmed W, Tariq S, Khan G. Tracking EBV-encoded RNAs (EBERs) from the nucleus to the excreted exosomes of B-lymphocytes. Scientific Reports. 2018;**8**:15438

[132] Moutsianas L, Jostins L, Beecham AH, et al. Class II HLA interactions modulate genetic risk for multiple sclerosis. Nature Genetics. 2015;**47**:1107-1113

[133] Hanisch U-K, Kettenmann H. Microglia: Active sensor and versatile effector cells in the normal and pathologic brain. Nature Neuroscience. 2007;**10**:1387-1394

[134] Voet S, Prinz M, van Loo G. Microglia in central nervous system inflammation and multiple sclerosis pathology. Trends in Molecular Medicine. 2018;**25**:112-123. DOI: 10.1016/j.molmed.2018.11.005

[135] Pender MP, Csurhes PA, Smith C, et al. Epstein-Barr virus-specific T cell therapy for progressive multiple sclerosis. JCI Insight. 2018;**3**. DOI: 10.1172/jci.insight.124714

[136] Cohen JI. Epstein-Barr virus vaccines. Clinical & Translational Immunology. 2015;**4**:e32